ABOUT THE AUTHOR

Lauren Callaghan (CPsychol, AFBPsS, PGDipClinPsych, PgCert, MA (hons), LLB (hons), BA) is a highly regarded clinical psychologist. She has worked at world-renowned research centres in London, UK, where she was recognised as a leading psychologist in the field of OCD, BDD and anxiety problems. Lauren received further qualifications in systemic family therapy and uses her expert skillset to work with individuals and their families to overcome obsessional and anxiety problems. After running a successful practice in London, she has recently moved to Sydney, where she continues to work as a clinical psychologist.

BY THE SAME AUTHOR

OCD, Anxiety and Related Depression
Body Image Problems and Body Dysmorphic Disorder

How to Help Your Child with Anxiety, OCD and Panic Attacks (2020)

LAUREN CALLAGHAN

HOW CAN I HELP?

8 WAYS TO SUPPORT SOMEONE YOU
CARE ABOUT WITH AN ANXIETY OR
OBSESSIONAL PROBLEM.

First published in Great Britain 2020 by Trigger

Trigger is a trading style of Shaw Callaghan Ltd & Shaw Callaghan 23 USA, INC.

The Foundation Centre

Navigation House, 48 Millgate, Newark

Nottinghamshire NG24 4TS UK

www.triggerpublishing.com

Text Copyright © 2020 Lauren Callaghan

British Library Cataloguing in Publication Data

A CIP catalogue record for this book is available upon request from the British Library

ISBN: 9781789561319

This book is also available in the following e-Book formats:

ePUB: 9781789561326

Lauren Callaghan has asserted her right under the Copyright, Design and Patents Act 1988 to be identified as the author of this work

Cover design by Bookollective

Typeset by Lapiz Digital Services

Printed and bound in Great Britain by CPI Group (UK) Ltd, Croydon CRO 4YY

Paper from responsible sources

DEDICATION

This book is dedicated to the tireless carers, partners and family members who love somebody with an anxiety or obsessional problem. Thank you for caring.

TABLE OF CONTENTS

INTRODUCTION

Thank you for picking up this book. You have probably selected it because someone you care for is suffering from an anxiety problem. From my perspective as a psychologist who has dedicated years to helping people recover from anxiety problems, your role is essential in helping your loved one get better. So, I want to thank you for being interested and caring enough to find out more about your loved one's problem and how you can help them.

I have written this book for you – for the families, partners, and/or close friends of someone suffering from anxiety. It contains advice and recommendations that I give to my clients and their families in my clinic, which they have found extremely helpful to know how to best support their loved one with an anxiety problem.

During my career I have become passionate about sharing knowledge and research-based treatment strategies with people. I trained as a clinical psychologist in New Zealand before moving to London in the UK. Whilst there I worked at the well-known Maudsley Hospital at research centres for anxiety disorders and trauma alongside diligent and world-renowned academics and clinicians who dedicate their lives to finding more effective treatments for these problems. I am grateful for my experiences working at the Maudsley Hospital and for my wonderful supervisors who imparted their knowledge and skills and ensured that my clinical work was up to their (very high!) standards. I specialised in Cognitive Behavioural Therapy (CBT) for anxiety and obsessional problems and I am passionate about improving access to these treatments for people who may not be able to access them in traditional formats of face-to-face sessions.

I have also always been interested in how our relationships and family networks interact with our wellbeing, because as people, we do not live in social vacuums. We exist in a system of people and this system can be of great benefit – as well as sometimes detrimental – to our health. Prior to working at the Maudsley Hospital I worked with young people and their families and I completed my postgraduate studies in family therapy. By combining my specialisms and interests, I hope to be able to improve the lives of people and make a positive impact with my work. I believe I am truly a better psychologist for my experiences of working with my clients and their families, and consequently I have been inspired to write self-help books for people – including families and partners of those suffering from mental health problems – who cannot easily access good quality help.

What I hope to achieve in this book is to teach you about anxiety and obsessional problems and how you can offer practical help to your loved one. The content is based upon the many appointments I have had with the families of my clients with anxiety and obsessional problems and the questions they have asked. I hope you find this book helpful, that you uncover things you didn't know already or learn new strategies that you have yet to try. And if you know it all already and all you take from this book is inspiration to try to help your loved one in a different way, then I consider it a successful outcome!

I have asked Alissa Shaw to co-write this introduction. I worked closely with Alissa, her husband Adam, and their children when Adam was suffering from a particularly acute episode of OCD. He had had OCD since he was a child but kept it in check to the degree that he was very successful in business and had a wonderful family. At the time I met Adam he was very unwell and the whole family was struggling to cope. Alissa was incredibly supportive of Adam but she needed some guidance on how to help him and what to expect during the treatment process. Adam eventually made a full recovery and, through his commitment to give back to the community, Adam and I co-wrote a CBT self-help book for people suffering from OCD and anxiety called *OCD, Anxiety and Related Depression – The Definitive CBT Guide to Recovery*. The idea was that through reading Adam's story, the reader would find the treatment more relevant. The feedback we have had is overwhelming and has inspired me to continue trying to help people via self-help books.

As Alissa has experienced many of the learning points and recommendations I outline in this book first-hand, she is the ideal person to share her story and provide assurances that these strategies do indeed work. I would like to thank Alissa for agreeing to share her personal experience below:

"To echo what Lauren has said, thank you for caring for your loved one with anxiety, and reading this book. As someone with first-hand experience of caring for someone with severe and crippling OCD, I know how tough, demoralising and incredibly stressful it is.

But I am happy to tell you that after undergoing treatment with Lauren, Adam got better. I had my husband back and our children got their father back. I hope you can relate to my story and that it gives you hope. Life can continue despite your loved one having a severe anxiety problem.

Our story started in Lanzarote in 2004. We went there to relax, unwind and enjoy a tranquil and slow-paced holiday, but it was a far cry from any of that. After a typical day by the pool, I went back to our house to find Adam lying on the bed in a teary, unintelligible state. Neither of us knew why.

Adam and I knew each other growing up and we share many sweet childhood memories. Our families were close and we took holidays together, sharing pizza evenings and going on family days out. We started dating when I was seventeen and Adam twenty-three.

I knew Adam incredibly well – or so I thought.

In truth, I didn't have a clue about his struggles with anxiety, which had been going on since he was a child. He simply kept it to himself, and he later explained that it was because he didn't understand what was happening to him. Keeping quiet was his strategy for carrying on with daily life. Adam has never had many outward or obvious OCD behaviours or rituals. His anxiety focuses on thoughts, and that's how he managed to hide it so often throughout his life. But on that day in Lanzarote, he could no longer keep the problem hidden. It was all about to come out.

My first instinct was fear. What in our lives could have been so bad that he ended up crying on the bed, feeling helpless and scared?

When he finally calmed down a little, Adam explained to me that he was terribly anxious. He'd been suffering for years, and now he could no longer make it go away. He just couldn't see an end to his distress.

Neither of us really had any idea about OCD back then. As with many people, I'm sure, the only knowledge I had about OCD was that it caused repetitive behaviours such as cleaning and hand washing, so OCD didn't even cross my mind. I presumed Adam was having some sort of mental breakdown, but I had no real understanding of the severity of the situation.

After we returned home to Sheffield and got back into a routine, things settled for a while. But as we would soon find out, this was just the beginning of our suffering at the hands of OCD.

It wasn't long before Adam fell apart again. We had a daughter together, and so it was very trying for all of us. We both worked, so when OCD struck again it was hard both logistically and emotionally. Adam could not go into work. He couldn't even leave his bed for a few weeks. He was so down and anxious; seeing him in that state devastated me. I just couldn't leave him alone – who knew what could happen? – so I was taking half days at work to get back home and make sure he was doing basic things such as eating and drinking. It was then that Adam saw a doctor and a therapist and got a diagnosis of OCD. Adam started using the therapy methods he had learnt, and they began to work. Thankfully it all felt as though it was working out. For the first time in a while, all seemed calm and hopeful.

In 2013 we went back to Lanzarote, this time to live there permanently. We were supposed to have a lovely, relaxed lifestyle there, but that didn't happen. Instead, there was more turmoil and devastation. Adam's OCD had returned... it seemed, with a vengeance.

He simply couldn't function. The strategies he learnt in therapy were no longer helping, and we soon found out that they had become part of the problem itself, a reassurance safety behaviour. And, as you will learn from this fantastic book, safety behaviours are an enemy in the disguise of a friend. He needed to get back to the UK and get more help.

The children and I stayed behind in Lanzarote while Adam went back to the UK to seek help. His mum came over to help me pack up our lives so that we could head back to England and help Adam get better there. This was one of the hardest rides of our lives – the worry and anguish was awful and the children missed their father so much.

Back in England, Adam was in a terrible place. For a week or so, I couldn't see a way forward. Adam wasn't getting better and I worried that maybe he was beyond help. Maybe this was how he would always be. Maybe we'd have to figure out some way of coping financially since he was unable to work. Maybe we would need to accept him like this and live with this illness forever.

My lowest point was when Adam suggested he admit himself to a place where he could stay and be cared for – such as a psychiatric hospital. The idea scared me. The truth was that I was struggling with the day-

*to-day workload of taking care of the children, taking care of Adam
and trying to stay upbeat and positive. It was exhausting.*

*It was at this point that a shining light came into our lives – in the
form of Lauren. Adam had researched some mental health charities
specialising in OCD and was given the name of some psychologists who
were known to be specialists in the field of anxiety and OCD. As I have
told her many times, I will be forever grateful to Lauren for giving us
back our lives, our future, our Adam.*

*During our very first visit she explained that yes, Adam did have OCD,
and no, it was not a life sentence. That he would recover. That moment
will stay with me until the day I leave this earth – there are no words to
describe how significant it was. I still get choked up thinking about it.*

*And so Lauren began teaching Adam how to overcome this period of
severe OCD. She also taught him how to live alongside the OCD, to not
just exist, but to live a fantastic life once again. And she taught me how
to help him do it.*

*This book would have been a lifeline for me and my family if we'd had
it when Adam was struggling with OCD. It would have been a welcome
resource to turn to every time I doubted my "help" for Adam. Knowing
that I was not alone in this and that there was hope for us would have
lifted my spirits and motivated me to change what I could to help him.*

*Adam made a fantastic recovery and we are now happy, healthy parents
to six wonderful children. Life has its ups and downs and we are
stronger together for having survived these episodes of OCD.*

*I sincerely hope that reading this book will give you the hope and help
you may need on your family's own journey and I wish you all the very
best."*

Alissa.

WHY SHOULD I READ THIS BOOK?

Anxiety problems are exhausting, time consuming, frustrating, emotionally draining and downright annoying. This applies not only to the person who is suffering from an anxiety problem, but also to you, the people who care for those individuals. No one opts to have an anxiety problem, just as no one wants someone they care for to suffer from an anxiety problem. Whilst there is a lot of help available for the person suffering from an anxiety problem, there is much less help available for their families, partners and friends.

In my experience during my years of clinical practice – especially those specialising in the treatment of anxiety problems – it is also families, partners and close friends who are in desperate need of guidance and support. You are the ones who witness and experience the actual impact of the anxiety problem and the real-time distress of the individual. I used to see clients for an average of fifty to ninety minutes a session per week, but families and partners were spending 168 hours a week living with the person, their anxiety problem and its associated burdens! (Admittedly, you may not be spending every second of the day with your loved one, but it will still be significantly more contact time than professionals.) And since you then need to add in all the complexities of family relationships, you are likely to be on call emotionally 24/7.

In fact, I saw many family members and partners who also became anxious and depressed because of their loved one's anxiety! And so I have written this book for you, the ones who are closest to those with the anxiety problems, to give you guidance on how to help your loved one and some practical tips to ensure you look after your own mental health.

A NOTE ON CASE STUDIES

Throughout this book, I have used case studies that are based on clients and families with whom I have worked. They are there to provide context or assist you when doing certain exercises. I have changed the names and small details in order to protect their anonymity, but I hope that you are able to relate to them and realise that your experience is more common than you think.

Is this book for me?

If you have picked this book up because of the title, then yes, it probably is for you. But just to be sure, ask yourself the following questions:

a) Does somebody close to you suffer from an anxiety or obsessional problem?
   That somebody could be anyone you are in a close relationship with – your adult child, parent, spouse or partner. It could also be a very good friend or someone else to whom you are closely connected.

   They could be suffering from a diagnosable anxiety or obsessional problem – such as obsessive compulsive disorder (OCD), panic disorder or social phobia – or they could be struggling with undiagnosed anxiety or worry. For the sake of clarification, obsessive compulsive disorders such as OCD and body dysmorphic disorder (BDD), are officially referred to in this book as "obsessional problems" although the sufferer experiences severe anxiety as part of the disorder. So, if I only refer to "anxiety problems" in this book, it includes obsessional problems too.

Anxiety problems are very common, with up to **one third** of people meeting the criteria for a diagnosable anxiety disorder during their lifetime and 2–3% of the population suffering from an obsessive compulsive disorder.[i]

Shona *has recently moved in with her boyfriend, Raj. They were dating for eighteen months before deciding to live together, and both are committed to having a future together. However, Shona is concerned that Raj's anxiety is becoming a problem. He has always seemed a bit stressed with work, but since moving in together Shona has noticed that Raj worries about a lot of things: work, money, future plans, his health... This impacts on his mood and sleep and Shona finds he is often quite negative about suggestions she makes. Shona loves Raj and wants the relationship to work out, but she would like him to see someone about his worries. Raj doesn't think he has a problem and is not receptive to seeking help.*

b) Do you sometimes struggle to know how to best care for your loved one?

It can be very difficult to know how to best care or communicate with someone who is suffering from an anxiety or obsessional problem. Their behaviour may be irritating, annoying, and downright strange. They may refuse to acknowledge the extent of their problem and the impact it has on other people. They may be accessing help and it may seem like nothing is changing, or they may refuse types of help such as medication or therapy.

Jon's wife, Evie, *has recently been diagnosed with agoraphobia. Evie is a primary school teacher but has been signed off work due to illness. She struggles to leave the house and won't go anywhere without Jon. Lately it seems like things have got worse, as Evie will no longer even go to the supermarket or to the local park for walks, which they did together. Jon wants* to support his wife, but he feels confused and does not know how to help her. The psychiatrist has said that she needs treatment, but she finds it too hard to leave the house to go for therapy sessions and she gets upset when Jon tries to make her leave the house. She takes an antidepressant prescribed by her doctor, but Jon doesn't think it has made any difference and is desperate for Evie to access more help.

c) Does your loved one's anxiety problem impact negatively on your life?

For example, do you change your plans for them, stop doing the things you enjoy, and make excuses for their behaviour? I have worked with many families and partners over the years who are all suffering in some way because of their loved one's problem. However, treatments are almost always focused on the individual who has been diagnosed with the problem, and not those who are supporting them.

Sue has a twenty-four-year-old daughter called Sara who has social anxiety disorder, which is getting increasingly worse. Sara was shy when she was young, and it became worse when she was a teenager. Sara has dropped out of college and moved home with her mother because of her problems. Sue finds it increasing difficult to know how to help Sara. She also gets frustrated and annoyed that Sara won't find a job and help out financially at home. Sue is feeling lonely herself because she no longer has her friends or extended family over at home for book club or dinner, as Sara finds it too stressful and Sue does not want to make things worse for her. But most of all, Sue worries about Sara and how to help her, and she just wants her daughter to be happy, engage in life and have a future to look forward to.

If you have answered "yes" to any of these questions, then this book is intended to help you. Anxiety and obsessional problems are extremely varied, and everyone's experience will be different, but the main thing is that everyone wants to help the people they care for to get better, and this book can help you be supportive in the right way.

You are **not** responsible for making your loved one better –
even if you think you are. *They* are! But you can be supportive
in a compassionate way and help them on their journey to
better mental health. Remember: it is no one's fault that your
loved one has an anxiety problem. But they can choose for
their future to be different and take steps to overcome the
problem.

Part of my treatment plan for individuals is to involve their
loved ones – usually the person or people they live with. Without
knowing it, your behaviour can unintentionally facilitate the
anxiety and obsessional problems, often allowing them to
become more entrenched, which is the opposite of what you are
intending to do!

This book will help you understand what drives anxiety
problems. I will explain the treatments that have been shown
to work and what families and partners can do to support their
loved one during treatment. It will help you to identify when you
can take an active role in the treatment process or when you need
to stand back a little bit and let the person take those steps on
their own.

I will talk about how to look after yourself in order to look after
somebody who is suffering from an anxiety problem, and provide
advice on how to communicate with somebody who is very
anxious or obsessional, as opposed to having difficult discussions
which then escalate into arguments.

Who isn't this book for?

This book is aimed at families and partners of adults with
anxiety and obsessional problems. I loosely define adults from
the age of eighteen and onwards, but if you have a mature

sixteen-year-old, then you may also find this book beneficial. It is **not** written for families with younger children and I would recommend that if you have a young child with an anxiety or obsessional problem, you should read my book for young people (*How to Help Your Child with Anxiety, OCD and Panic Attacks*).

It is also not written specifically for people who are suffering post-traumatic stress disorder (PTSD), which occurs following a traumatic experience. PTSD requires a particular treatment which I do not discuss in this book. However, PTSD can be present alongside anxiety and obsessional problems. If this is the case, the advice in this book will still be helpful and relevant for you.

Also, if your loved one is severely unwell and you are worried about them hurting themselves or that they may try to commit suicide, then please seek help immediately. If you are worried about upsetting them, you can sort that out later once they have received the help they need. It is more important that they get the help to keep them safe; you can work on relationship upsets once your loved one is more settled.

What if my loved one has depression or another mental health problem as well?

It is very common for people suffering from an anxiety or obsessional problem to also experience low mood or clinical depression. If you consider how much the mental health problem is sabotaging their life and preventing them from living the life they want, then it is no wonder that they may also be depressed. If they are, then it is still okay to use the techniques in this book. In Part Two, Chapter 8, I look at depression in further detail and provide suggestions on how you can help your loved one if they are suffering from depression as well.

However, it can also be the case that the depression is so severe that it will stop your loved one from being able to get better, as they may feel it is pointless or they may lack the energy or motivation to engage in treatments. If this is the case then I strongly recommend that you encourage them to get the depression treated first, as it will be too difficult to undertake any other active treatments, even if they want to overcome their anxiety and/or obsessional problems.

It is also very common for anxiety problems to co-occur alongside mental health problems other than depression, including personality disorders, eating disorders, neurodevelopmental problems such as autism, and other types of anxiety disorders.

If your loved one is suffering from another mental health problem as well as anxiety or obsessional problems, this book is still for you – though if your loved one has another mental health problem, the treatment of the anxiety or obsessional problem will likely take longer than the standard course of treatment. This is because the "standard" treatment is based upon people who have only one anxiety or obsessional disorder without other complicating factors. However, the good news is that they should still make improvements with treatment and have a better quality of life.[ii]

CHAPTER SUMMARY

- If someone you love has an anxiety problem, whether it has been formally diagnosed or not, it can be difficult to know how to best care for them and support them.
- Despite anxiety and obsessional disorders being very common, it is still difficult to find helpful advice about what you should (or should not) be doing to help your loved one.
- It is likely that this person's anxiety problem is impacting negatively on your life, perhaps without you even realising it.

- Anxiety problems co-occur with a lot of other mental health problems including depression and other anxiety disorders, but this does not stop treatments from being effective and you can still use the strategies in this book.
- If your loved one is very depressed, it could be hard for them to engage in treatment for their anxiety problem, so it may be best to have the depression assessed and treated first.
- It is no one's fault that the person you love is suffering from an anxiety problem, but you are also not responsible for making them better. They are responsible for getting better, but you can support them along the way.

PART ONE

UNDERSTANDING ANXIETY AND OBSESSIONAL PROBLEMS AND THEIR EFFECTS

CHAPTER ONE
WHAT IS ANXIETY?

Whilst I'm sure you have googled "anxiety" and read what you can on the topic to better inform yourself, people I see in clinic like to have their understanding of anxiety corroborated by an expert. They also want to know when it is considered a "problem" as opposed to normal worry and stress. Here I will briefly review the fundamentals of anxiety and then cover the specific diagnosable anxiety and obsessional disorders.

So, what exactly is anxiety?

Anxiety is a very human condition. It is an interplay of your thoughts, emotions, physiology and behavioural responses. Everyone experiences anxiety to some degree. It's a normal reaction to something you perceive as a threat. For example, if you believe you are being followed on your way home at night, you are likely to react cognitively, emotionally and physiologically. Your emotional reaction may be one of fear. Physiologically, you may start to sweat and shake and feel your heart rate increase. Your cognitive response is to think you are in some form of danger. No matter that the person could just walk past and pay you no attention; you have responded instinctively to what you perceive as a threat.

Anxiety is a normal human reaction to something you perceive as a threat.

Anxiety has a pretty impressive physiological reaction. When you perceive a threat, your body responds by releasing the neurochemicals cortisol and adrenaline. Cortisol is a steroid hormone that is produced by the adrenal glands which sit on top of each kidney. Adrenaline is another hormone that is produced by both the adrenal glands and a small number of neurons in the base of your brain. Both these hormones play an important role in the fight, flight or freeze response. More cortisol in your system gives you quick bursts of energy for survival and lower sensitivity to pain. Cortisol also curbs functions that are non-essential or unhelpful in that moment, such as suppressing your digestive system. Adrenaline makes your heart beat faster and your lungs breathe more efficiently. It causes the blood vessels to send more blood to the brain and muscles, increases your blood pressure, makes your brain more alert, and raises sugar levels in the blood to give you energy to either fight or flee.

Fight, Flight or Freeze

When you first perceive a threat there are three choices: fight, flight or freeze. Do you wait until the person reaches you and fend them off? Do you freeze on the spot and wait for them to pass? Or do you run away from danger? Fight, flight or freeze is an evolutionary response from prehistoric times that has (very usefully) stayed with us. It is an innate, protective response which keeps us safe. Of course, this response makes more sense when the threat is obvious, such as a large teeth-baring animal running towards our ancestors – a prowling sabre-toothed tiger, for example. However, as we have developed as humans and become more sophisticated and complex in the way we live, it is often harder now to identify what a "threat" really is. Today, threats are not just physical; they can be mental and emotional too. So, while our threat system still operates as it did with our ancestors, it can be much trickier to pin down the actual threat.

For example, the threat of losing your job could cause you as much anxiety, relatively speaking, as the sabre-toothed tiger did to our cavemen ancestors. Although this threat doesn't mean you will die, there is the threat of losing income which may result in debt, financial hardship for your family, loss of status, the struggle to find a new job, etc. And all that is, of course, a threat to your survival in today's world.

When does anxiety become a problem?

Think about a time that you have felt anxious or fearful – did you notice any of the following physiological symptoms?

- Increased heart rate
- Jumpy or easily startled
- Sweating
- Feeling hot
- Dry mouth
- Nausea or upset stomach
- Tense muscles
- Narrowed vision (tunnel vision)

These are all common symptoms of the fight, flight or freeze response. You could experience some of these while watching a scary movie on TV or in anticipation of a significant event like a job interview, first date, or an exam. I would be surprised if you cannot recall a single time when you experienced the physiological changes of anxiety in your body. Because, as

I repeat, anxiety is a normal human condition and we all experience it, even the most outwardly calm among us.

People like your loved ones, who experience anxiety in a problematic way, will have the same physiological symptoms as those above – although they will experience them more frequently and more acutely. In fact, there is good evidence that experiencing chronic anxiety – i.e. being in the fight, flight or freeze physiological state more often, and for longer periods – and the overexposure to cortisol and other stress hormones can disrupt almost all your body's processes. This puts people at increased risk of many health problems including depression, digestive problems, headaches, heart disease, sleep problems, weight gain and memory and concentration impairment.[iii]

Anxiety is normal, but it can become misplaced or misdirected. It becomes a problem when you experience it too frequently and/or intensely and your appraisal system isn't managing it as well as it should. This happens when you misinterpret something as a threat, estimate the risk of the threat disproportionately (in that it is more likely to occur) and believe the consequences of the threat will be disastrous.

The term "anxiety" covers the full range of anxiety presentations and symptoms, from minor symptoms – such as being worried that you will be late for an appointment or meeting – to severe anxiety, which manifests itself in an actual disorder like panic disorder, social anxiety or OCD. When you have anxiety that is interfering significantly in your work, personal or social

---

Anxiety problems occur when you misinterpret things as threatening and interpret threats as much riskier than they actually are.

The words "stress", "worry", "fear", "panic", "keyed up" and "on edge" are used in relation to everyday occurrences but these terms – and many others – all refer to anxiety.

life, it is likely that you have an anxiety or obsessional "disorder". These are conditions that mental health professionals agree are best represented by a cluster of symptoms that we use to help diagnose somebody and offer suitable treatments.

Not all people who experience problematic anxiety will meet the criteria for a diagnosable mental health disorder, but they may find that their symptoms interfere with living and enjoying life. Consequently, you, as their family, partner or close friend will also experience interference in your life in some way. Most likely you will also experience conflict or distress in your relationship with the person who has the problem.

So if anxiety is stopping the person you care for engaging and enjoying life, it is likely they have a diagnosable anxiety disorder.

Why do people get anxiety problems?

This is the big question, and if we knew exactly who was going to develop an anxiety problem, then we could probably make an intervention earlier to prevent it becoming problematic! The truth is that we do not know who will develop an anxiety or obsessional problem, despite anxiety being one of the most common mental health problems. We know that one in three people experience problematic anxiety at some time in their life, and estimates are that one in five people currently have an anxiety or obsessional problem. Also, women are twice as likely as men to have an anxiety problem. So that's a lot of people (and women in particular) suffering from problematic anxiety.[iv]

Whilst we don't know exactly what causes these problems, we believe it is likely a to be a combination of genetic, psychological and environmental factors. Some disorders are triggered by a specific event at any age, whilst others start in childhood. There is no one pathway for anxiety or obsessional problems, but we know that they can become severe and chronic if the person doesn't get the right help.

I often had family members, particularly parents, ask me if they were in any way responsible for causing their loved one's problem. The answer is no, you are not. Even if you contributed genetic material, there are still other factors that cause an anxiety or obsessional problem. If it was just genetic, then everyone sharing the same genes (all siblings) would develop the same mental health problem, and this does not happen. So we know there are other mediating factors at play. There may well be things that you do that contribute to the ongoing anxiety problem without realising it, but I will talk you through these in later chapters. But rest assured that you did not cause your loved one's anxiety problems.

Jennifer's eighteen-year-old son Tre has contamination OCD – the type where he worries about germs and catching an awful illness if he touches "dirty" things. This includes anything touched by people outside the house – e.g. all clothes, food and money. Tre has become housebound and spends a lot of his day engaged in cleaning and decontamination rituals. Jennifer worries that she somehow caused Tre's OCD – she always kept the house very clean and told her children when they were little not to touch things she considered dirty. Jennifer has two other sons aged sixteen and twenty-three and neither of them have anxiety or obsessional mental health problems.

Panic attacks

People often use the term "panic" or "panic attack" to describe an anxious state, but it does not always mean they are referring to an actual panic attack. When mental health professionals refer to "panic attacks" we are referring to a specific instance in which a person's anxiety symptoms are physically overwhelming but last for a fairly short time.

A panic attack is described as "an abrupt surge of intense fear or intense discomfort that reaches a peak within minutes". During that time, four (or more) of the following symptoms can occur:[v]

- Palpitations, pounding heart, or accelerated heart rate
- Sweating
- Trembling or shaking
- Sensations of shortness of breath or smothering
- Feelings of choking
- Chest pain or discomfort
- Nausea or abdominal distress
- Feeling dizzy, unsteady, light-headed, or faint
- Chills or heat sensations
- Paresthesias (numbness or tingling sensations)
- Derealisation (feelings of unreality) or depersonalisation (being detached from oneself)
- Fear of losing control or "going crazy"
- Fear of dying

You can expect panic attacks in situations you fear, or they may occur out of the blue. For example, you may have a panic attack at a public speaking event if you have social anxiety disorder, or you may have one unexpectedly when walking down the street. They can happen any time during the day or night. Regardless of whether they are predictable or not, they are scary and distressing and can make you want to avoid any situations that you believe may bring them on. Panic attacks can also occur as a single one-off event or as a feature of another anxiety problem. For example, if you suffer from OCD or a phobia you may experience panic attacks as part of that problem. Or you may just have one panic attack in response to a single event and it never reoccurs. Panic attacks are also a main symptom of panic

Panic attacks are a normal human experience, but they can become problematic if they occur too frequently or in the context of a diagnosable anxiety problem.

disorder, a specific anxiety disorder in which you worry about having panic attacks.

Panic attacks are very common, and people without anxiety problems can experience them too. I still recall having a panic attack when I was at college and had an assignment due. I had stayed up most of the night and had drunk a lot of coffee. In the morning I was walking to college to hand in the assignment and about halfway there I had a panic attack. It was very unpleasant and scary, and I wasn't sure what was happening, so I sat down and waited until it passed. I (helpfully in hindsight) interpreted it as a reaction to having very little sleep and drinking far too much coffee. I was not in graduate training then, so I didn't know what it was – although knowing what I know now, it was clearly a panic attack. Had I interpreted it as a very scary event, in which I might collapse or die, or that I was going crazy, then I would likely have worried about it happening again and be on my way to developing an anxiety disorder! Whilst I am grateful that it didn't escalate into anything problematic, I can say it was a very overwhelming and frightening experience – one that has stayed with me.

CHAPTER SUMMARY

- Anxiety is a normal human reaction and we all experience it.
- Anxiety is a reaction to something you perceive as a threat and it is an interaction of your thoughts, emotions, physiology and your behavioural responses.
- Fight, flight or freeze is an evolutionary response which enables our bodies to react to a threat.
- Anxiety becomes problematic if it is experienced too frequently and in situations that are non-threatening or present a very low level of risk.
- Whilst anxiety disorders are some of the most common

mental health problems, we cannot predict who will develop one, although it is likely to be a combination of biological, genetic and psychological factors.

- Panic attacks are specific surges of intense and debilitating anxiety which reach a peak within minutes. They can occur any time and can be part of a specific anxiety disorder.

CHAPTER TWO
ANXIETY AND OBSESSIONAL DISORDERS

In this chapter I describe the different anxiety and obsessional disorders. I will give you some examples of people I have treated with these types of problems and the impact of their illness on the people around them. Behaviours (the outward presentation of the problem – the part you are most likely to see) can be extremely varied in each disorder, and in some cases I have provided two case studies to highlight this. The impact on loved ones will also vary depending on the severity of the problem. Some people with an anxiety problem may be able to leave the house, continue in a job and support their dependants; others may be housebound and spend most of the day worrying about things or spending excessive time on seemingly pointless rituals.

Anxiety and obsessional disorders are grouped according to a common set of symptoms that are backed up by academic research. Because anxiety and obsessional disorders are organised by clusters of symptoms, many symptoms overlap and people often meet the criteria for more than one anxiety disorder at a time. For example, someone with social anxiety disorder may also meet the criteria for generalised anxiety disorder, and someone with OCD may also meet the criteria for body dysmorphia (BDD). Each disorder has a specific psychological treatment and it is possible that if your loved one meets the criteria for more than one anxiety or obsessional problem, they may need to have more than one course of therapy.

Anxiety disorders

An anxiety disorder is defined as a condition that causes people to experience "excessive fear and anxiety and related behavioural disturbances".[vi] Specifically, fear is the emotional response to real or perceived imminent threat and is associated with the physiological changes in the body for the fight, flight or freeze response. Anxiety is the anticipation of future threat and is accompanied by increased muscle tension and scanning the environment in preparation for future threats. However, the terms "fear" and "anxiety" overlap a lot and are often used interchangeably, so don't worry too much about whether you are using it correctly. For your purposes of understanding anxiety problems and helping yourself and loved ones through them, it doesn't matter which term you use.

In anxiety disorders people experience fear in situations which have a low level of threat. This means they are either misinterpreting a situation as threatening or overestimating the likelihood of the threat occurring. Consequently, this results in changes in their behaviour – avoiding the threat or trying to reduce the chance of it happening. So, the fear and anxiety they experience is disproportionate to the situation, and the way they respond is unhelpful. In fact, it often ends up feeding into the problem.

If someone meets the criteria for one anxiety disorder, it is possible that they will meet the criteria for another anxiety disorder.

Despite having a common group of symptoms, an anxiety disorder can still vary widely on presentation, frequency, and severity.

GENERALISED ANXIETY DISORDER (GAD)

People with GAD may be described as "worriers", which makes sense as GAD is defined by excessive and uncontrollable worry for reasonably long periods of time. Whilst everybody worries some of the time, in GAD it is the *uncontrollability* of the worry – people cannot switch off from it, stop it or distract themselves from it – and the *amount* and *length of time* they worry that causes a problem. To be diagnosed with GAD, people must worry more than half the days in a week for more than six months. The worry can jump from subject to subject and can lead to worry about worry itself. For example, someone with GAD may worry that *"if I keep worrying likes this, I will cause myself serious health problems"*. People experience physical symptoms of anxiety including restlessness, irritability, muscle tension and sleep problems. Sufferers may have had GAD for many years, but usually only seek help or get formally diagnosed when they are in their thirties.

June is a fifty-six-year-old woman who worries all the time about everything and anything – from taxes, to her health, to whether she made the right decision at the shops. She has always been a "worrier" and June doesn't remember a time when she wasn't worried about something. It is exhausting. She finds it hard to sleep and often has tension headaches. She had hoped that once her two sons had grown up and left home, she may worry less about them, but in fact it feels like she is worried more than ever since they left home. Her sons do not know how to help her and now call and visit less frequently. They wish she would talk to someone and get some counselling and stop calling to check on them all the time.

SOCIAL ANXIETY DISORDER (SOCIAL PHOBIA)

This is when people fear how they will be scrutinised or judged in public. It can apply to any situation where a person feels "on show" and at risk of being negatively judged by others, for example eating, social events or meeting new people. People try to find ways to minimise their anxiety, including avoidance of the situations and other counter-productive behaviours. For example, someone worrying that other people find them boring or dull, might drink too much alcohol at a party to feel more relaxed and confident and to stop themselves worrying so much, but ironically this makes them worry more the next day because they can't clearly remember what they said or how they acted. Social anxiety disorder is most likely to start in teenage years, with the average age of onset being just thirteen years old![vii]

Mo is eighteen. He has always been painfully shy and since finishing secondary school he has become even more introverted. He now spends most of his time at home on his computer, writing code for people who contact him online. Mo's parents are beside themselves with worry as he rarely leaves the house and hides away in his room when they have visitors. Every time they try to talk to him, he gets angry and withdraws back into his room. His parents are also arguing a lot over the best way forward for their son and both are feeling very stressed.

Raj is a thirty-six-year-old business consultant. He has a partner and they have an active social life, enjoying attending dinner parties and trying new restaurants with friends. Raj has had social anxiety since college. He hates public speaking and being in groups with new people and finds that he becomes very anxious. Raj has managed his anxiety relatively well with medication and cleverly being able to avoid most anxiety-producing situations. His partner, Sasha, finds it frustrating, and does not like making excuses for Raj. They do fight about Raj's anxiety occasionally, particularly after evenings socialising when Raj keeps asking Sasha whether he said or did anything stupid when they were out. Most of all, Sasha just wants Raj to feel more confident and stop criticising himself after social events as she hates seeing him down or distressed.

Phobias

A phobia is an intense fear of a specific object or situation, such as snakes, spiders, flying or open spaces. The way people respond to the object or situation is excessive and disproportionate to the actual threat and may cause the person to avoid everyday things or situations. Although some phobias may be more common, you can in fact develop a phobia about anything. However, a phobia, like all mental disorders, must cause significant impairment in one area of your life.

Interestingly, blood injury phobia is the only phobia in which people are likely to faint or pass out. People do not usually faint in response to fearful situations, as their blood pressure increases due to their heart rate rising in the fight, flight or freeze response. In order to faint your blood pressure needs to drop, but when you are anxious your blood pressure rises and your heart rate increases. Therefore, fainting in the context of anxiety peaks does not happen – despite what TV shows might try to tell us. We don't know exactly why people faint in blood injury phobia, although it has been suggested that it has an evolutionary cause.[*]

Stephen *is twenty-eight and has a phobia of flying. This isn't much of a problem in his day-to-day life, but it causes a lot of conflict in his family as he will not fly for family events or holidays. His sister recently got married and he opted for an eleven-hour coach ride rather than a quick ninety-minute flight after work to attend her wedding. Whilst Stephen has managed to avoid it so far, he really would like to fly, especially now his girlfriend Sarah has moved to England for work. Sarah wants Stephen to come and visit, but he is worried about flying. Sarah is very frustrated and thinks Stephen should get some treatment and then visit her. She is thinking of ending the relationship as she doesn't want to be with someone who doesn't seem to want to better himself or try to overcome his phobia for her.*

Joan *is thirty-two and has recently married Pierre, whom she had been dating for three years. She and her husband were very happy and did not argue much until recently when they discussed starting a family. Joan suffers*

[*] It is thought that if there is blood, especially if it is your blood, it would be advantageous to lie down and slow down your pulse so the blood stops pumping so fast, thus losing less blood. Also, if blood is spilled, then it may be best to play dead (i.e. faint), so any blood-thirsty enemy would ignore you.

from emetophobia, a phobia of vomiting, and avoids anything that she thinks might make her likely to vomit. This includes long-distance travel, types of food and drink, visiting ill friends (or friends with young kids, as we all know that they get sick all the time!), amusement park rides, and any other activity where she might vomit or be exposed to people vomiting. Pierre is very keen on starting a family, and although Joan wants children, she does not want the nausea and morning sickness associated with pregnancy or little children throwing up at home. The issue is starting to dominate their time together and every conversation ends up in an argument about Joan's phobia. Pierre believes that if Joan really wanted to get over her phobia she would, and he is starting to really resent the impact it is having on their lives.

PANIC DISORDER

This is when people experience panic attacks that cause them to worry that they will lose control of themselves or be harmed in some way, for example having a heart attack or a mental breakdown. While panic attacks are common in all anxiety and obsessional disorders, in panic disorder the fear is, in fact, one of having more panic attacks. The person goes to great lengths to avoid situations in which they worry they could have a panic attack.

Ralph is twenty-three and is a keen amateur runner. However, he has started getting panic attacks and he worries that he is going to lose control of his bowels when he is away from home. This means that he no longer goes on training runs and makes sure that he is close to home or an accessible toilet whenever he leaves home. Ralph is paying a lot of money to get taxis to work as he worries that he may need to go to the toilet when he is on the bus between stops. Ralph has also stopped going out with his friends as he is so worried that he will have another panic attack and need the toilet urgently. His roommates are worried that Ralph is becoming depressed, as he hardly leaves the flat unless it is to go to work. His best friend John is very worried about him and does not know what to do. Ralph is too embarrassed to talk to anyone professional, but John wants his friend to be happy and get his life back.

AGORAPHOBIA

People with agoraphobia are incredibly fearful or anxious of two or more of the following:

- Using public transport (e.g. buses, trains, trams, airplanes)
- Being in open spaces (e.g. car parks, arenas, bridges, parks)
- Being in enclosed places (e.g. shops, theatres, cinemas)
- Standing in line or being in a crowd
- Being outside of the home alone

People with agoraphobia worry that they will not be able to escape or access help if they start panicking or think they will have a panic attack. Women are twice as likely as men to suffer from agoraphobia, and whilst most people are diagnosed before the age of thirty-five, you can develop agoraphobia at any age.[viii]

Olga is thirty-seven and has two children. She has panic disorder and agoraphobia and is now housebound. She lives with her parents after separating from her husband because she cannot afford her own place, nor can she cope on her own now. She worries that she will go mad or lose control of her actions in some way and may not be able to escape from the situation she is in. This is having a very negative impact on herself, her children and her parents. Her parents take the children to school and to their sport events, do all the shopping and other jobs requiring leaving the home. They do not understand Olga's problem and are getting fed up with the situation. They love having their grandchildren around and being involved in their lives, but they have their own physical health issues and have recently retired from work. They want Olga to get some help for all their sakes.

Other types of anxiety problems

If you do not think your loved one has one of these anxiety disorders but still experiences problematic anxiety, there are other categories of anxiety problems.

UNSPECIFIED ANXIETY DISORDER AND OTHER SPECIFIED ANXIETY

"Unspecified anxiety disorder" is when someone has an anxiety problem that does not meet criteria for any particular disorder. "Other specified anxiety disorder" covers anxiety that is problematic and similar in nature to an anxiety disorder, but does not meet the *full* criteria for the anxiety disorder. For example, a person could have what feels like panic attacks but with only two or three symptoms of a panic attack (you need four to meet the full criteria of a panic attack). They could have generalised anxiety but only worry less than half the time (in the criteria it specifies "worrying more than half the time"), but they still could find it difficult to control and have problems sleeping and relaxing. Like the other anxiety disorders, someone suffering from "other specified anxiety disorder" must experience significant impairment in some way due to the anxiety.[ix]

There is also a category called "substance/medication-induced anxiety disorder" in which people experience panic attacks or anxiety in response to being intoxicated or withdrawing from a substance, medication or a toxin. This is likely to resolve once the person has stopped using the substance or medication or stops being exposed to the toxin. Another category is "anxiety disorder due to another medical condition" in which a person suffers anxiety or panic attacks due to an underlying medical condition. A number of medical conditions are associated with increased anxiety including respiratory illness, neurological problems, metabolic disturbances (such as low B12), endocrine disease (including hyperthyroidism) and cardiovascular diseases. The anxiety symptoms will often reduce when the medical condition is treated effectively. However, anxiety disorders can develop in their own right following or alongside medical problems, so it is very important to get a diagnosis from both your medical doctor and a psychologist and get a combined treatment plan – particularly if both the health condition and anxiety disorder require treatment and medication.

Obsessional Disorders

As I mentioned, OCD and similar obsessive problems are not formally categorised as "anxiety disorders", despite one of the main symptoms being anxiety and that they were once considered part of the anxiety disorders spectrum. They belong to the obsessive compulsive spectrum of disorders in which people experience obsessions and/or compulsions.

Just to be clear, this book is also written for people with a loved one suffering from an obsessive problem. Like anxiety problems, obsessive problems can vary considerably in their severity and presentation. I have worked with people who were treated successfully for their OCD in under ten sessions as well as people who were completely housebound and dependent on their families and therefore required much more intensive treatment.

OBSESSIVE COMPULSIVE DISORDER (OCD)

OCD is a problem that can be about anything, manifesting itself in unwanted, intrusive thoughts, urges or images ("obsessions") which are recurrent and persistent, combined with repetitive behaviours or mental acts ("compulsions") intended to deal with or avoid such obsessions. For example, intrusive thoughts about becoming contaminated with bacteria may lead to time-consuming and over-the-top hygiene practices, including excessive handwashing and showering.

You may be familiar with the representation of OCD on TV and films, but this is not usually very sophisticated and can perpetuate unhelpful stereotypes of OCD. TV often depicts germ obsessions and cleaning or washing compulsions and rituals. If your loved one is suffering from OCD, then you are probably aware that OCD can be about anything – not just germs! – and usually involves concerns of causing harm or damage to someone or something (obsessions), being held responsible for that harm or damage,[x] and trying to stop it from happening (compulsions).

Although the specific content of obsessions and compulsions varies among individuals, certain types of obsessions are more common in OCD, including those of cleaning (contamination obsessions and cleaning compulsions); symmetry (symmetry obsessions and repeating, ordering, and counting compulsions); forbidden or taboo thoughts (aggressive, sexual, and religious obsessions and related compulsions); and harm (fears of causing harm to oneself or others and related checking compulsions).

Jordan is twenty-three and lives at home with his mother and stepfather. the focus of his OCD has changed over the years, and has now become centred on whether he has inadvertently caused an accident somehow, such as knocking a cyclist off their bike while driving or leaving an appliance on at home. He obsesses about whether he really wants to cause an accident or hurt someone, and whether this makes him a terrible person. He has stopped driving and avoids leaving the house. He constantly checks with his family members whether he has caused an accident, watching the news to check up on accidents that he might have been responsible for. His mother and stepfather are very concerned and think that he may need to be hospitalised. They also don't know how to talk to Jordan about this problem because every time they approach him, he breaks down in tears and tells them he thinks he is crazy.

Cynthia is thirty-two and lives with her husband Robert and their two daughters. She has had OCD for as long as she can remember, although she has kept it in check and been able to live her life unfettered by it. However, following the birth of her second daughter, Cynthia's OCD has got worse and she now worries about germs and bringing a terrible illness into the house that would infect her children or husband. She has started cleaning for hours at a time and now washes everything that she believes is not clean enough. She makes her children and husband shower immediately after being *outside and spends a lot of money on disinfectant wipes and other cleaning products. Robert is concerned about her and the effect it is having on the family. He hates seeing Cynthia distressed, but is getting sick of having to shower after taking the rubbish bins out or collecting mail. He is also worried about the impact of her behaviour on their daughters. He isn't sure who to turn to for help and what the next steps should be, but he knows that they cannot continue as they are.*

BODY DYSMORPHIC DISORDER (BDD)

In BDD a person worries excessively about one or more slight or perceived defects in their appearance that are not noticeable or appear very insignificant to others. They then perform repetitive behaviours and mental acts in response to their worries and they camouflage, hide or disguise the perceived flaw. For example, someone who worries that their facial pores may be too big may check their appearance obsessively in the mirror, wear heavy make-up to cover them, hide behind scarves and hats, seek unnecessary and often expensive cosmetic procedures, and constantly compare their skin to that of other people.

Jayne is a twenty-year-old student and has suffered from BDD since she was sixteen. She worries about her skin pigmentation and she spends at least two hours a day applying make-up and dressing or arranging her hair to hide her skin. She refuses to have photos taken and will not sit in brightly lit areas. Her boyfriend, Jay, does not understand her problem as he believes she is beautiful. He gets annoyed that she won't let him post photos of them on Instagram and is bewildered by her behaviour. Recently Jayne has become more distressed and she spends days in her student room without leaving. Jay is worried, frustrated and confused by her behaviour and does not know how to talk to her about what is going on.

Viktor is twenty-four years old and works as a plumber. He lives with his aunt and uncle and has a close-knit family. Viktor is worried about having excess fat on his stomach. He works out every day and eats a protein-rich diet. Viktor believes that he has more fat than he should and that it looks funny and he is convinced people will notice. He wears loose-fitting clothing and avoids swimming, showering at the gym, and intimacy. Viktor would love to have a girlfriend but is worried that she would notice what he believes is a major flaw in his appearance. His family know that Viktor is worried about his looks, but they don't know specifically what he is concerned with as he is too embarrassed to talk about it. His aunt would love Viktor to be more confident and start dating and she wants to know how to best help Viktor.

There are also other "related" disorders under the obsessive compulsive disorder heading: hoarding, trichotillomania (hair pulling) and skin excoriation disorder (dermatillomania or skin picking). These are not traditionally known as "anxiety" problems because they are considered "compulsive" problems in which a person will feel compelled to act in a certain way. If your loved one is suffering from one of these problems, they will need a specific psychological treatment for that disorder, but a lot of the advice in this book will still be helpful for you.

HOARDING DISORDER

You may be familiar with people who find it hard to throw things out; in fact you might be one yourself! However, hoarding disorder relates to more severe presentations – like the ones often broadcast for reality TV. I watch these with a lot of empathy for the individual and their families; having worked with people with severe hoarding disorder, I know how distressing and embarrassing these problems are for the sufferer. Hoarding disorder is when people can't discard things, regardless of their cost, as they believe they need to save them. This becomes problematic when possessions clutter up the home and it becomes unlivable.

TRICHOTILLOMANIA

Otherwise known as hair pulling disorder, trichotillomania is when someone repeatedly pulls out their hair and cannot seem to stop despite trying hard to do so. Trichotillomania results in hair loss to varying degrees which can cause further distress to the individual.

EXCORIATION DISORDER

Otherwise known as skin picking or dermatillomania, excoriation disorder is when someone keeps picking their skin despite efforts to stop. It often results in visible skin lesions, which can be embarrassing or distressing for the individual.

Other types of obsessional disorders

UNSPECIFIED OBSESSIONAL DISORDER AND OTHER SPECIFIED OBSESSIONAL DISORDERS

Similar to anxiety disorders, there are other categories of obsessional problems. "Unspecified obsessional disorder" is when someone has obsessive problems but does not meet the criteria for a particular disorder. There is also the category of "other specified obsessional disorders" which covers obsessional problems similar to OCD and BDD, but do not meet the full criteria of that disorder. This includes obsessional jealously – which is where someone is obsessed about their partner's perceived infidelity – or body dysmorphic obsessions in which the person has a noticeable flaw in their appearance (as opposed to BDD when the flaw is slight or doesn't exist).

Similar to the anxiety disorders, there is a category called "substance/medication-induced obsessional disorder" in which people experience OCD-like symptoms in response to being intoxicated or withdrawing from a substance, medication or a toxin. It is likely to resolve once the person has stopped using the substance or medication or stopped being exposed to the toxin. This is very rare and often only occurs in the case of stimulants (including cocaine), or heavy metals and toxin poisoning. The last category is "obsessive compulsive and related disorder due to another medical condition" where a person suffers OCD-like symptoms due to an underlying medical condition. There is some controversy around whether some OCD and related problems can be caused by certain streptococcal infections, but to date there is not enough evidence to suggest a causal link. Although, in some cases, OCD-like symptoms can arise after a stroke.

HEALTH ANXIETY

The official term is "illness anxiety disorder"; however, psychologists and doctors are likely to label it health anxiety. It comes under the category of "somatic symptom and related disorders",[xi] but in the DSM-5 (the bible of mental disorder categorisation[xii]) it is acknowledged that illness anxiety disorder could also be considered an anxiety disorder. It is very similar to OCD, in that someone obsesses about their health and falling ill in the absence of physical symptoms or very minor physical symptoms. The associated compulsions include checking their body for signs of illness, seeking reassurance via frequent visits to the doctor or, increasingly now, self-diagnosis on the Internet.

George is forty years old and lives by himself but has a very close circle of friends with whom he meets up regularly. George has had anxiety problems for a while, but recently this has become focused on health issues and whether he has an underlying neurological illness. George worries he may have MS or Lupus and is constantly checking his body for signs of nerve damage. He googles symptoms that he is experiencing and has visited his doctor and other specialists multiple times. He can barely sleep and has stopped seeing his friends and family. George's friends do not know what to do; they don't understand what is happening for George. They know he is worried about his health but can't understand why he isn't listening to the doctors when he is told that he is very unlikely to have one of these illnesses. They feel drained and frustrated that their reassurances don't seem to be making any difference.

Maria has become convinced that the fillings she received in her teeth when she was a child may be toxic and poisoning her. Despite several dentists reassuring her that this is extremely unlikely, Maria is not convinced and has spent a lot of time researching the subject. She has found a dentist who will remove her teeth, for a cost. Maria's sister Ava, who is her key support, is alarmed – she believes it is an extreme response to remove eight teeth and is trying to talk Maria out of this surgery. Maria is incredibly anxious and convinced this is the only way to feel better. Ava wants Maria to stop being so anxious and obsessive. She is sure there is another way to help her, but finds all conversations are circular and come back to Maria wanting the surgery.

A NOTE ON "INSIGHT"

As clinicians we use the term "insight" to record how much a person recognises they have a mental health problem and require help to overcome it. It is useful because it helps us choose how to start a psychological treatment and what type of therapy would be most helpful to start. For example, someone with social anxiety disorder may recognise they have an anxiety problem and that they require help which would show "good insight", and they would be given an active therapy – Cognitive Behavioural Therapy (CBT) – to directly treat their disorder.

However, someone else with BDD could be adamant that they do have a problem with their appearance and that they do not have a mental health problem. They would be considered to have "poor insight" into their problem and we would provide them with a therapy designed to help them see they have a problem first. In this instance the psychological treatment may be Motivational Interviewing, which is a talking therapy designed to help people overcome ambivalence towards changing their behaviour.

CHAPTER SUMMARY

- Anxiety and obsessional disorders are problems which can be diagnosed by a professional and are defined by a cluster of symptoms.
- Anxiety disorders are defined by excessive fear in response to a situation that is non-threatening, or situations in which the likelihood of risk is very low.

People with anxiety disorders then avoid the situation or develop safety behaviours designed to reduce the risk and lower their anxiety.

- In obsessive compulsive disorders people experience persistent and uncontrollable obsessions which can be thoughts, images, doubts, fears, impulses and worries. They also engage in repetitive behaviours or compulsions to minimise the threat of these obsessions and to reduce their anxiety.
- Even if your loved one doesn't meet the criteria for a specific disorder, they can still have an anxiety problem and may have an "unspecified" or "other specified" disorder.
- An anxiety or obsessional disorder can vary considerably in its presentation and severity.
- "Insight" refers to the level of acceptance that a person has about their mental health problem and helps guide the type of talking therapy that could be offered.
- Illness anxiety disorder, or health anxiety, is another type of anxiety disorder in which someone worries obsessively about their health.

CHAPTER THREE
COMMON FEATURES OF ANXIETY AND OBSESSIONAL DISORDERS

Whilst it is all well and good understanding the classification of anxiety and obsessional disorders, it can sometimes be hard to translate the diagnostics into your own reality and I hope you may have been able to relate to some of the case studies along the way.

Below are some of the common features that are seen with anxiety and obsessional problems. I have no doubt you will recognise some of them.

Common Features

RUMINATION

Rumination is a "mental behaviour" in which someone attempts to deal with upsetting events by thinking about them over and over again in an unhelpful way. People focus on past experiences and think about how they would have done something differently which may have prevented a particular outcome from happening. Everyone does this and it's completely normal, but it becomes a problem when you can't stop it and feel more anxious and down because you can't stop thinking about upsetting things.

For example, Jane has social anxiety disorder and recently at a work lunch she stuttered over a couple of words and found it difficult to speak when she was asked what she did over the weekend. She felt so embarrassed and has since thought about the event non-stop and how she should have responded – without stuttering. She has found it difficult to focus on her work or sleep at night. People who ruminate a lot can be described as "being in their heads" and appearing distracted by the internal dialogue. Rather aptly, the word "rumination" comes from "ruminate", which is what cows do when they chew the cud over and over and over again. It's a great description of the process of people chewing things over in their heads.

WORRY

Worry is very similar to rumination, and it can be hard to separate the two. But I use the term "worry" to describe the mental process of focusing on things that may happen in the present/future, whereas rumination is usually focused on past events.

THINKING PROBLEMS

Both worry and rumination involve what I call "thinking problems" – unhelpful patterns of thinking. You will probably identify with some of the thinking problems, but rest assured, everyone engages in these ways of thinking. It becomes a problem when you get stuck in them, and they make you feel anxious and down and cause you to behave in counterproductive ways.

Here are some of the more common thinking problems seen in anxiety and obsessional problems:

- **Catastrophising** – thinking the worst-case scenario about every event, no matter how minor.
  My loved one will never recover from this problem.
- **Thought-action fusion**[xiii] – having such a thought means it is more likely to happen, or it means that thinking about the action is as bad as actually doing it. This is very common in OCD problems.

I had a thought about hurting people and that is just as bad as actually hurting someone.

- **Magnified duty**[xiv] – believing you are 100% responsible or have an increased responsibility for things, discounting the fact that other people may also share responsibility.
  I must make sure everyone is packed for the camping trip tomorrow as I organised it.
- **Personalising** – thinking that everything is your fault, even when you couldn't have had anything to do with it.
  It must be my fault that my partner doesn't want to get help with his anxiety problem.
- **Black-and-white thinking or all-or-nothing thinking** – experiences or things are only categorised as one way or another, often as good or bad, with no in-between.
  I didn't do well in my therapy session today so the whole treatment must not be working.
- **Crystal ball thinking/forecasting the future** – thinking you can predict the future or living as if the future has happened.
  I have to spend my whole evening preparing for this meeting tomorrow as I just know I will be asked a difficult question.
- **Jumping to conclusions** – making a judgement, usually negative, even when there is little or no evidence for it.
  I know that my colleagues think I am boring if I don't tell exciting stories at lunch.
- **"Should be" and "ought to be"** – thinking things HAVE to be a certain way, or people (including you) SHOULD behave in a particular way.
  I should be feeling better by now as I have had five sessions of CBT treatment.
- **Guarantees about the future** – needing everything to be guaranteed or the outcome of events to be known, despite this being impossible.
  If I go shopping, I need to know that there will be no queues and there will always be a toilet close by.

- **Emotional reasoning** – basing things on how you feel, rather than reality.
  I feel really anxious, therefore there must be something I am worried about that I haven't sorted out yet.

  Perceived control or superstitious thinking – believing you have control over events or outcomes that you cannot actually influence. This can sometimes be known as "magical thinking" in its extreme form.
  If I plan this outing in detail, I can prevent anything unforeseen happening.
- **Overestimation of likelihood or possibility** – believing an event to be imminent and extremely likely to take place despite how unlikely it is in reality.
  If I don't check the door to make sure it is locked, someone will definitely break in.
- **Mind reading** – believing that you know what other people are thinking, despite having no evidence for it.
  I know everyone will think I am stupid if I give this presentation and don't know all the answers.

OBSESSIONS

Obsessions are persistent and uncontrollable thoughts, images, doubts, fears, impulses and worries. These are also known as intrusions because they've suddenly intruded on your everyday thinking. In the case of OCD, obsessions are usually related to causing harm in some way, and in BDD they are about a perceived defect in appearance. They will be made up of at least one "thinking problem". For example, someone obsessing about their appearance in BDD will catastrophise the outcome, overestimate the likelihood of something happening, believe they know what others are thinking (mind reading), and jump to conclusions, e.g. *everyone will notice that I have a huge forehead and think I am so ugly. It will be so embarrassing; I won't cope and I will have to leave immediately.*

AVOIDANCE

Avoidance is a fairly obvious feature of anxiety and obsessional problems. If you are scared and worried about something, you will do your best to avoid it. In fact, this makes perfect sense. But in the case of anxiety or obsessional problems avoidance becomes problematic, with people often taking drastic steps to avoid their feared event. Also, avoidance actually reinforces the original problem. For example, if you are anxious about going to the dentist, your *catastrophising* belief of this event is that it will be painful and unpleasant, and you won't cope with the pain and anxiety of being there. However, if you have a toothache and you avoid the dentist, the physiological consequence is that it will become worse, perhaps requiring more serious treatment at a later stage. In addition, your avoidance has stopped you disproving your belief that it will be painful and unpleasant and that you would not cope, thereby actually giving more weight to your original (and likely untrue) belief about going to the dentist!

SAFETY BEHAVIOURS

Safety behaviours are actions carried out by people in order to feel safe from their worries or prevent a feared outcome. They can take any form and include avoidance, mental rituals, mantras, compulsions, and rituals. They can be very obvious or they can be cleverly disguised in other forms. For example, someone with a phobia of dogs may plan their route from home to the shops in detail to avoid any dog walkers or parks. Someone with BDD may be so concerned about their nose that they wear excessive amounts of make-up and large scarves to cover it.

COMPULSIONS

Compulsions (including rituals) are a type of safety behaviour that occur in the obsessive disorder spectrum of disorders. They are actions that people feel driven to do in response to an obsession. They are used to minimise or prevent the threat of the obsession and to reduce the person's anxiety. They are usually repetitive behaviours such as switching light switches on an off, counting to a certain sequence, or monotonous cleaning or washing behaviours. Compulsions can include mental behaviours (or mental rituals) too, such as repeating phrases or mantras or undoing "bad" thoughts or images with "good" ones. Compulsions can take many forms; I have seen some very creative and unusual ones, including walking backwards while retracing steps home from my clinic!

REASSURANCE SEEKING

This behaviour is where someone seeks reassurance that something bad hasn't happened or won't happen. It can take many forms, including asking family and friends, searching online, and seeking advice from professionals. For example, someone with health anxiety may seek reassurance from their partner, their doctor, specialists, or Dr Google. Ironically, seeking reassurance actually makes people worry more rather than abate their worries. The person with health anxiety will probably feel better shortly after seeing a doctor, but then start to worry that they hadn't explained the problem properly or that the doctor missed something, and then will start worrying all over again. And the reassurance received will never be enough – they will come back for more. It is a bit like a short-acting mood-enhancing drug – in the short term it helps and feels good, but it will soon wear off and you will be back at the same place you were before you took the drug, and therefore will take it again to feel better, and so on, and so on…

SHAME AND EMBARRASSMENT

Pretty much everyone I have ever seen in clinic with an anxiety or obsessional problem is ashamed and embarrassed about their problem. They do their best to hide it and are usually reluctant to talk to people – including their loved ones – about the problem or aspects of it. This is not surprising – people are usually well aware of how irrational their worries can be, how unreasonable their behaviour becomes, and how demanding it can be on their loved ones. However, in the throes of an anxiety problem, a person feels so anxious and finds this so unbearable that they will continue to do anything they can to not feel that way, including their unhelpful behaviours. For example, someone may have OCD and experience intrusive thoughts about behaving in a very inappropriate, sexual way. They may be afraid of what this means about them and obviously worry that someone will find out and believe they are sexually deviant or dangerous, therefore they will be unlikely to disclose these worries to anyone, even to their nearest and dearest. (I have seen this type of OCD in my clinic countless times! It is quite common but very scary and unsettling for the clients and their families.) So please keep in mind that any reluctance to talk to you about their problems is often down to shame.

SELF-CRITICISM

Similarly, people suffering from anxiety and obsessional problems are very self-critical. They blame and criticise themselves for having the problem and not being able to overcome it on their own. They criticise themselves for any situation that they did not handle "perfectly", which results in anxiety. A common way to try to change others' behaviour is to point out what they are doing wrong, but this is not likely to be effective as people who are self-critical are already beating themselves up. So be mindful that if you try to point out what is wrong with your loved one's behaviour, they probably know it already and are already punishing themselves.

LOW SELF-ESTEEM

Not surprisingly, people who suffer from anxiety and obsessional problems who experience a lot of shame and self-criticism suffer from low self-esteem. They often believe they are weak, worthless and undeserving. This is another reason why a punishing or critical approach doesn't help to get them motivated or change their behaviour, as they may believe they deserve to be criticised and punished and that they do not deserve to get better.

SELF-MEDICATION

This is another common feature of anxiety and obsessional problems. With self-medication, people take a substance without medical advice with the intent of lessening their symptoms and emotional distress. This includes alcohol, cannabis, over-the-counter medication and other substances. It can also be considered a safety behaviour and like other safety behaviours it is counterproductive and often ends up making the anxiety worse. I would commonly hear from my clients with social anxiety that they would drink alcohol at social events to feel less inhibited and to reduce their worries and anxiety, and whilst this worked at the time, the morning after they would experience more severe anxiety and worry about whether they behaved inappropriately. They would also worry because due to the alcohol, they would not remember clearly what they actually did. Not to mention that alcohol can also be a depressant – it negatively affects mood – which doesn't help when one is feeling hyper-anxious with a hangover.

ASSOCIATED DEPRESSION

I have already mentioned that people with anxiety and obsessional problems are more likely to suffer from depression as a result. The obvious impact of this is that people may feel less motivated, more fatigued and more hopeless about getting better. I will talk about this more in Part Two, Chapter Eight, but I have included it here to remind you that some of the reluctance or inability to get help may also be as a result of depression.

SECONDARY GAINS

Sometimes people can get additional benefit from having an anxiety or obsessional problem which we refer to as a "secondary gain". For example, they may not have to do boring but necessary tasks (such as supermarket shopping or cleaning) and they may get a lot of sympathy and attention from other people. Sometimes family members have complained to me that their loved one is "putting it on" or is "lucky to get out of chores" or that they "love" the attention they receive. It is true that some people receive a type of benefit for having an anxiety or obsessional problem, but I want to be clear that it is very rare that someone would want to stay unwell due to these "gains". These secondary gains are usually time limited and do not compensate for the severe anxiety and length of illness that someone experiences.

CHAPTER SUMMARY

- *Rumination* is when people focus unhelpfully on the past, whereas *worry* is about future events.
- Everyone experiences thinking problems, but in anxiety and obsessional disorders thinking problems can become stuck and people struggle to see situations any other way.
- Avoidance is very common in anxiety and obsessional problems as people will understandably seek to avoid anxiety-provoking situations.
- Most people with anxiety and obsessional problems will perform safety behaviours which are designed to minimise the perceived threat and reduce their anxiety, although safety behaviours are counterproductive and end up reinforcing the problem.
- Some people may experience secondary gains as part of their anxiety or obsessional problem, but these are

---

unlikely to compensate for the distress they experience or prevent them from getting better.

- People with anxiety and obsessional problems are more likely to experience depression, low self-esteem, and self-criticism. They are also likely to feel ashamed and embarrassed about their problem.
- People may self-medicate with alcohol and drugs to minimise their anxiety and distress, which can be problematic and can further entrench the problem.

CHAPTER FOUR
THE IMPACT ON YOU

I have no doubt that your loved one experiences distress and a reduced quality of life due to their anxiety or obsessional problem. But for now, let us turn the focus onto you and your family or dependants and think about how your loved one's problem affects you all. It is likely that you and other family members are experiencing a reduced quality of life too – especially if you have to deal with things such as constant underlying concern about your loved one's wellbeing, physical demands (e.g. time-consuming rituals) placed on you, extra work to support your family (financially or otherwise), constant reassurance seeking, or having to pick up the slack. When you add in having to make excuses for your loved one's behaviour or absence and the time taken away from socialising, relaxing or leisure activities, the sheer emotional drain of caring for someone with an anxiety or obsessional problem is enormous.

It doesn't matter whether your loved one has a problem which is triggered in specific situations (e.g. a phobia), a chronic problem that is longstanding, or a recent onset of a problem which is severe. The onset and pattern of these problems can vary considerably, and it doesn't really matter what it looks like, because it still has a very strong impact on people around them.

Emotional impact

Think about the effect your loved one's problem has on you emotionally. How do you feel because of your loved one's problem now and how do you feel about it in the moments when it is at its peak? Or when you are asked to do things that you don't want to do, such as partaking in a ritual, making excuses, or give reassurance for the thousandth time?

Below are all feelings that families and partners have told me that they feel in response to their loved one's anxiety or obsessional problem.

- Frustrated
- Annoyed
- Sad
- Angry
- Resentful
- Anxious
- Embarrassed
- Irritated
- Irate
- Down or depressed
- Defeated
- Disappointed
- Devastated
- Overwhelmed
- Ashamed
- Fearful
- Hopeless
- Exasperated

You will note that they are all what you may experience as unpleasant emotions,* but I have yet to meet someone who tells

* I believe it is not helpful to label emotions as "good", "bad", "negative" or "positive" because this then leads to the idea that we should not experience "bad" or "negative" emotions, whereas it is part of life to experience a range of emotions. I prefer to use the term "unpleasant" to describe what may otherwise have been referred to as "negative" feelings.

me they feel happy or excited or positive about their loved one's anxiety problem.

You will of course feel more uplifting or pleasant emotions such as relief, hope and happiness when your loved one seems to turn a corner and is open to receiving help or is on the path of recovery. However, it will still be a rollercoaster of emotions as there will be periods of setbacks and difficult parts of treatment that cause more anxiety (I know this is precisely what they are trying to avoid experiencing and I will explain this in more detail in Part Two, Chapter Four). But at this point rest assured that what you are feeling is NORMAL and it is okay to feel all the things you are feeling yourself. It does not mean that you care for your loved one any less. Acknowledging how you feel and knowing that is okay will help you know when you need to have some time away to rebalance and when you will be more effective in helping your loved one with their problem.

Jayne and Fez *have a twenty-five-year-old son called Trevor. Trevor has OCD. He obsesses about whether he will hurt someone and whether this makes him a psychopath. He has had OCD for seven years and it waxes and wanes – sometimes it is severe, leaving him housebound, and other times he is able to live a fairly normal life. Jayne and Fez are exhausted and worried about his future. Every time he says he will get help they feel relieved and hopeful, but as soon as the symptoms reduce, he says he does not need help as he "has it under control". Jayne and Fez then feel despondent and down, and when Trevor's OCD becomes problematic again, they become anxious, annoyed and angry. Fez is also starting to feel depressed and Jayne thinks he needs help for his low mood. What a rollercoaster!*

Behavioural impact

Families and partners always change their behaviour in some way either to accommodate their loved one's anxiety problem or to minimise their distress. This is a very normal thing to do.

Whilst you may make only minor changes initially, if your loved one's problem goes unchecked then any changes you make will become more extensive and start interfering in your enjoyment of life or ability to do important things.

There may be many things that you no longer do that you used to. It is important to acknowledge what these are and why you are not doing them, as the reasons are likely to vary. There may no longer be time to do them or you may be too tired because you have to take on other tasks. You may feel guilty about having fun or doing anything for yourself. Maybe you feel overly responsible for your loved one or worry about what other people think about you leaving them alone when they have an anxiety problem.

Take a moment to think about the things that you do or don't do to accommodate your loved one's anxiety or obsessional problem? These could be work, social or leisure related, or extend to household maintenance and chores. What is the reason you are not doing these things? It can be helpful to ask yourself these questions and note down your answers.

To help you think about this, I have provided a case study below.

Joseph's wife Nurima has GAD. She is not sleeping well and is feeling fatigued. They have a one-year-old baby and Joseph is getting up early to look after him and get him ready for the day before going to work. He also comes straight home after work to help his wife and do the household chores. Joseph obviously doesn't mind as he wants to support his wife and family. He is a keen runner and hasn't been able to find the time to run recently. Running helps him feel happier and balanced and he misses it.

He feels responsible for his family and he believes it would be selfish of him to go running when his wife is suffering from anxiety. He is also not going to Friday night work drinks with his colleagues anymore. His mood is flat and he has put on weight.

Joseph's list:

I no longer ...

Go running or meet my work colleagues on a Friday.

Why do I no longer do these things?

I feel guilty leaving my wife alone as she is not coping very well.
I am tired as I am doing all the household chores and looking after our son, as well as working full-time.
I don't seem to have the time now as I am busy all the time looking after our son.

What effect is it having on me?

I feel down now myself. I have put on weight which makes me feel worse and I haven't had a chance to debrief from work which I used to find helpful.

Now write your own answers below.

I no longer...

Why do I no longer do these things?

What effect is it having on me?

Giving reassurance

Reassuring people you love is a very normal thing to do, and it is okay to do it in the absence of an anxiety or obsessional problem. My sister often asks me for reassurance on the psychological aspects of parenting, such as setting behaviour reward plans for her children. This is fine as it happens once or twice a year and I feel good for helping her. However, if she was ringing me a couple of times day asking me for reassurance on whether she was doing the right thing with the reward charts, I would undoubtedly become frustrated that she wasn't listening to me and taking my advice – not to mention the time it would take up in my day that I couldn't then spend on more helpful or enjoyable activities. It would then negatively impact my mood and make me snappy and irritable with my family. I would start thinking of ways to avoid taking her call, which would take up more mental space and distract me from the tasks I need to complete.

One way of thinking about the impact of giving reassurance is to think about it in terms of time, namely the time it is taking away from other more enjoyable or necessary pursuits. I have provided a case study below as an example of how to do this.

Kiera is married to Julian, who has social anxiety disorder. He worries about how he comes across at work and in other social situations. Julian will often text or call Kiera during the day to seek reassurance on social interactions, sometimes up to six or seven times on a particularly anxious day. By the time Keira has thought about it and responded, each call or text takes approximately five minutes. Then at home in the evening Julian details his interactions and asks for her advice and reassurance. This takes around thirty minutes. Then, if they have a social event in the evening, he will seek reassurance afterwards or the following morning (fifteen minutes).

Without realising it, Kiera has spent over an hour on average per day just on reassuring Julian. That's seven hours per week, twenty-eight hours per month, and 336 hours (a full two weeks!) per year!

And that is just for the reassurance side of things! This doesn't even factor in the time it takes to plan social events that Julian feels comfortable going to, time giving excuses for events that he does not feel he can attend, and time coaxing him to try new events. Nor does it consider the time spent turning around and going home after setting out to social occasions. That could total another seven hours a week – which in total is one full month a year accommodating Julian's social anxiety. That is a lot of time that could be spent elsewhere! Kiera could write a book, train for a marathon, study or complete a training or education course... You get the picture. And if you are completing rituals for someone in case of OCD, you are quite possibly spending even more time on these too.

How much time does your loved one's problem take up in your life? Fill in the table below. I appreciate these are just approximations and different factors will impact on this. However, this is to help show you that it is likely taking more time from you than you thought it was.

	TIME TAKEN UP ON REASSURANCE:	TIME TAKEN UP ON OTHER THINGS (MAKING EXCUSES, PLANNING SOCIAL EVENTS, GOING HOME EARLY OR EVEN *BEFORE* AN EVENT):
DAILY		
WEEKLY (X7)		
MONTHLY (X4)		
YEARLY (X12)		
GRAND TOTAL:		

When you realise how much time your loved one's problem is taking up, you may start feeling (even more) resentful and angry towards them. At this point, it is useful to think of your loved one's anxiety problem as *separate* to them. You can then direct your anger and resentment towards the anxiety problem, not them. It is not their fault they have this problem; it is the anxiety or obsessional problem causing them to feel and behave this way. However, they can still take responsibility for getting better and they may require some support and help with that (which is why you are reading this book).

Impact on children

Family members often worry about the effect of their loved one's disorder on children. If you have children with someone who has an anxiety or obsessional problem, then you have most likely seen the impact on them. Depending on the age of the children, they may see that Mum or Dad behaves in funny ways, or "doesn't feel right", or "doesn't like" specific things or places. Children are very astute and pick up on emotional cues quickly. They may not have the words to describe what is going on, but they notice things aren't right.

They may think, *why does Mummy always check the windows and doors?* Or, *why is Daddy feeling sad?* Children also learn by *modelling* (copying) behaviour they see. My one-year-old takes tissues and wipes my nose and tries to wipe up mess under her highchair (very unsuccessfully) only because she has seen me do this, not because she was born with an innate sense of hygiene and cleanliness. As children grow, they model your behaviour in all types of environments. For example, if you have a phobia about dogs and every time you pass a dog when you are out with your children you startle and move away, your children will notice and take home the message that dogs are dangerous.

So, even despite best efforts, children will know when one of their parents has an anxiety or obsessional problem. They may not understand the details of the problem, depending on their age and comprehension ability, but they will know something is going on and is not okay. I recommend that you find a way to talk to your children about what is going on so that they have some guidance and they know it is okay to ask you questions. By far the most helpful thing is for children to see their parent who is unwell overcome their problem, as this models bravery, courage,

---

Modelling is when a person observes the behaviour of another and then imitates the behaviour.

---

determination, and success – and who doesn't want their children to be exposed to those qualities?

The majority of people I see in clinic are well aware of the potential impact of their problem on their children. They worry about the example that they are setting, feel guilty for not being able to parent in the way they would like, and are ashamed of the problem. Having children can be a great motivator to get better from an anxiety problem, so instead of using the impact of the children as a criticism, it would be better to use it as a positive motivator.

CRITICISM:

'Can't you see the impact this is having on the children?'
'You are a terrible role model!'
'You don't seem care about the children.'

MOTIVATION:

'The children love you and you need to get better to give them the time and attention they deserve.'
'You can be a good role model to the children – you have a problem and can choose to overcome it, no matter how hard it is.'

'You love the children and owe it to yourself to be the parent you want to be.'

I have also had expecting parents frequently ask me whether they would pass on their anxiety problem to their children. If you are thinking of starting a family with someone with an anxiety or obsessional problem, there is no clear link that genetics alone causes these problems as they are believed to arise from a combination of genetics, environmental and social factors. There is no guarantee that your child won't have an anxiety or obsessional problem, but there is no absolute causation that has been proven. In addition, your child would also receive half of your genetic material too, will grow up in a different family and environment to your partner, and will be exposed to your protective and resilient behaviour. So there are a lot of differentials to ensure they will not be a carbon copy of your partner and inherit their anxiety problem.

Neglect

Whilst child neglect is not usually caused by anxiety disorders, in rare cases parents with OCD can experience problems in caring for their children. If someone has intrusive thoughts about causing harm to their children, they will start avoiding doing things they think could lead to harm, for example bathing them. It can be an unintended consequence of an OCD safety behaviour too – if someone worries about causing an accident when driving, they may avoid driving altogether, which is very problematic if they have to drive their children to school every day and have no other way of getting them there.

However, to be clear: just because someone has intrusive thoughts about children or causing harm to them, does not mean that they are a danger to children! If anything, the opposite is the case, as the person is so worried about the content of their thoughts that they will avoid any situations with children. I have lost count of the people I have treated for OCD who had intrusive thoughts about children, and not one of them has posed any risk to children. It is only a risk when people are in positions of caring for children and the thought of harming them repulses them so much that they become unable to properly care for them. If you are concerned that your loved one is unable to look after their children properly, then you need to contact help immediately (social services, your loved one's doctor or psychologist, or emergency services).

Susan has three children aged one, three and six. She has OCD and is currently experiencing a severe episode in which she worries about harming her children. She has intrusive thoughts about drowning them in the bath, poisoning their food or smothering them at night when they sleep. Susan loves her children dearly and is horrified at these thoughts; she worries she might harm them without knowing it. To make sure this doesn't happen, she no longer bathes them, makes them food, or puts them to bed or down for naps. Her husband John has now realised the extent of the problem and has had to take a lot of time off work and ask friends and family to help out.

Impact on sex life

If you are in an intimate relationship with someone with an anxiety or obsessional problem, then it is very likely you will have problems in your sexual relationship.

It can be difficult to be in the mood for sex when you are frustrated, angry and resentful at your partner and having more arguments than usual. It could be that due to the anxiety and depression – or the medications they're taking – your partner has a reduced libido and does not feel like having sex. If your partner has BDD, it may be that their body concerns are getting in the way of intimacy. If your partner has OCD, it is possible that their obsessions are about bad hygiene during sex, or they may have intrusive thoughts during the sex itself, which puts them off as they worry about having further thoughts during sex.

So, anxiety and obsessional problems can affect intimate relationships in a lot of ways. Intimacy is an important part of a relationship and it helps you feel connected with your partner. It also provides health benefits and helps your mood. Even without sex, actions such as touching, hugging, kissing or sitting with each other watching a movie hand in hand are ways of being physically close. These activities can all be affected if your partner is in the throes of an illness.

It can also be very difficult to talk about intimacy and sex, especially if you feel you're going to upset your partner or cause additional stress. So at this point I encourage you to think about your intimate relationship and whether it is being affected by their anxiety and obsessional problem. What was your physical relationship like before the problem or when the problem was less severe? What would you like your physical relationship to be like in the future?

By thinking about intimacy and labelling it a problem (if it is indeed a problem), you are providing space for things to improve. It may take some time and require some further conversations, and perhaps your partner has to receive help for their anxiety and obsessional problem first. But it may be that you can create space for more intimacy if your partner starts receiving help for their problem. You can create a plan for yourself to address this either now or in the future, and make sure you check in with yourself in six months to see if things have changed (hopefully for the better).

Take a moment and consider the following questions for yourself:

- If a lack of intimacy or sex is a problem for me, what, if anything, can I do about this now?
- Is this something that I can speak to my partner about now?
- Can I be more affectionate and make time to be physically close with my partner?
- If not, is this something that I can mention is a problem that I would like to address in the future?
- What steps can I take to address this now or in the future? (E.g. self-help books, speaking with a relationship therapist.)
- Can I set a reminder in my phone or on my calendar to check in on this issue in six months?

Anxiety or depression

Are you suffering from anxiety or depression as a result of your loved one's problem? Let me reassure you that this would not be uncommon. I have worked with many partners and parents of people with anxiety or obsessional problems who had become depressed or anxious as a result of living with their loved one's problem. It is not surprising when you have to accommodate someone else's anxiety or obsessional problem in your life and all the demands it makes on you. It also may be that you have an underlying anxiety problem that has been triggered by your loved one's anxiety problem.

If you have found yourself feeling down for the past two weeks, have lost interest in things you used to enjoy or are not getting as much pleasure from them, you could be depressed. Please read through the list of symptoms on the opposite page and tick any that apply to you.

Over the past two weeks, which of the below have you experienced?
- Feeling down, sad, or depressed
- Loss of interest or pleasure in things
- Significant weight loss or gain
- Changes in appetite
- Problems sleeping
- Fatigue or loss of energy
- Slowness in thoughts or in bodily movements
- Feeling more agitated
- Feelings of worthlessness or excessive guilt
- Difficulty in concentrating or thinking
- Indecisiveness
- Thinking about suicide, or planning suicide

If you tick more than three of these boxes, I would recommend seeing a mental health professional for your own assessment. There is absolutely no shame in being depressed; it is not your fault and it is understandable given how stressful things have been. It is important, however, that you seek help. You cannot support your loved one in their journey to get better if you are not well. It is also very good modelling behaviour if you receive help with your mood. It may encourage your loved one to seek help too.

Julia and Hugh's twenty-one-year-old daughter Kim suffers from BDD. She barely leaves her room, let alone the house, and if she plans to go out, she spends hours putting on clothes and make-up, before deciding she no longer wants to go out. She gets very distressed when people come to the house, so Julia has stopped having friends over. Julia is worried about Kim and has noticed that she herself is feeling hopeless about Kim's future. As a result, her mood is very low. Julia doesn't see her friends very often and can no longer be bothered going to her spin classes, which she used to enjoy. She works part time, but recently has been calling in sick. She also has much less of an appetite and has stopped cooking family meals. Hugh thinks Julia is depressed and wants her to see her doctor, but Julia thinks it is just stress from worrying about Kim and thinks that after a few nights of good sleep, she might snap out of it.

It could be that you have only developed an anxiety or mood problem since dealing with your loved one's anxiety – though it is very unlikely to be caused directly by their anxiety problem.

It is very important, though, that you receive treatment for your own problem so you can continue to support your loved one.

It may be that you need medication, or perhaps self-help treatments or a course of good therapy will help.

The "silver lining" here is that you will be able to undertake the experiments part of treatment (that I discuss later in this book) alongside your loved one.

You need to be healthy and mentally well to be able to best support your loved one in their journey.

CHAPTER SUMMARY

- A person's anxiety or obsessional problem affects those around them, especially partners and family.
- You will experience a lot of emotions, most likely unpleasant ones. This is very normal.
- You are likely to change your behaviour in a way that you believe helps your loved one, but in fact contributes to the ongoing problem.
- You may be giving your loved one reassurance in some form, which is also unhelpful and keeps the problem going.
- If you have an intimate relationship with someone who has an anxiety or obsessional problem, it is common to experience problems with maintaining a sexual relationship.
- Children will be impacted if they are in close contact with someone with an obsessional or anxiety problem, but you can help manage this by talking to them and explaining what is going on.
- It is extremely rare for cases of child neglect to be caused by anxiety or obsessional problems, and it will most likely occur in the context of OCD obsessions about causing harm to children.
- You may become depressed or anxious as a result of living with your loved one's problem, so please get some help and look after yourself so you can provide the support your loved one needs.

CHAPTER FIVE
HOW YOU ARE PART OF THE PROBLEM

Problems do not occur in isolated environments. They are the products of different factors interacting with each other. This is true of anxiety and obsessional problems too, as they also occur in a multifaceted environment clouded by complex human relationships and interactions.

Without meaning to, humans can often have a negative effect on those around them, and this is very true in the case of anxiety and obsessional problems. This is not intentional and often we are not even aware that what we are doing is unhelpful. And even if we are aware, we may find it difficult to change our responses. So the purpose of this chapter is not to blame you or criticise how you respond to your loved one, but to help you reflect on how you are responding and whether you are able to change some of the things you do.

We all respond in unhelpful ways under pressure sometimes. Even as a psychologist my responses are not perfect – my family will certainly attest to that – but I try to learn from my behaviour, and improve the way I respond. Remember, the goal is to facilitate positive change for your loved one, and if by changing the way you respond you make that more likely to happen, then that is a win-win situation.

HOW ANXIETY WORKS

Let's start by looking at a model of an anxiety problem.

The trigger event is the precursor to the worry or obsession. It can be a place, person, situation, future event, body sensation or even a thought itself! For example, in the case of social anxiety disorder, the trigger could be a scheduled work social event that causes this worry: *I will say something stupid and everyone will notice.* In the case of a phobia, it could be the specific thing you are afraid of – a snake, a dog, or a spider, for example.

With OCD the trigger could be a thought, image, urge, desire or action, for example an intrusive image of germs infecting your family which then leads to obsessions about hygiene and cleanliness. It could be something that is on the TV, read in the newspaper, or said in a conversation. A trigger can be anything that then causes you to worry. It doesn't really matter what it is though, as you cannot change triggers – they will continue to occur whether you want them to or not.

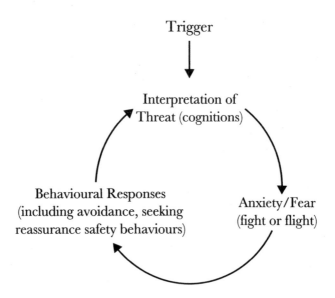

A trigger then leads to the "actual worry" which is the (mis) interpretation of a threat. This is the cognitive process in anxiety and obsessional problems – the thing that is going through your head. So, in the case of the work social event, it would be the thought, *I will say something stupid and everyone will notice*. In the case of a phobia it may be *dogs are very dangerous* or *flying is a very unsafe way to travel and planes crash all the time*. In the case of OCD, it may be *I have had a thought about my family dying from illness and that means it is really likely to happen*. If you recall from earlier, these thoughts are when you misinterpret events as threatening or believe the threat as much more likely to occur than it really is.

Not surprisingly, when you interpret something as threatening or believe there is likelihood of harm, you feel panicked and anxious in your body. This physiological reaction is the fight, flight or freeze response kicking in.

The behavioural response is what action you take as a consequence of this "threat" as your body is in fight, flight or freeze mode and is now telling you that you need to react to the threat. I have referred to these responses earlier as "safety behaviours" and this is where we find all sorts of expected and unexpected responses. It makes complete sense to avoid things that you believe may present a threat or to try to mitigate the threat in some way. It also makes sense to seek reassurance that the threat will not occur or, if it does, will not be as awful as you expect.

So this all seems pretty reasonable in the face of a threat, right? However, remember, in the case of anxiety and obsessional problems the threat does not exist – or if it does, the likelihood of it occurring is minimised.

In the case of social anxiety disorder, if the threat of social rejection is very real then it makes sense to minimise that threat by avoiding social situations or seeking reassurance that you have behaved appropriately – remember, to our ancestors, social rejection would have meant certain death if they were exiled from their community. But we know that when someone has social anxiety disorder, they perceive social threats when they are not present. And if the threats *are* present (and let's be honest, pretty much all social interactions come with a possibility of rejection), they believe that bad things are definitely going to happen and the results will be disastrous.

Therefore, all safety behaviours are pointless because the threat either doesn't really exist or is extremely unlikely to occur. Mind you, if you try to tell someone suffering from an anxiety or obsessional problem that their behavioural responses are futile, it is unlikely to go well. You have probably done that anyway and know the outcome!

So, these behavioural responses continue to reinforce the message that there is something dangerous to avoid or manage, and therefore lead back into the original worry. This is known as the vicious cycle of anxiety and obsessional problems. It becomes a stuck loop which feeds on itself. Imagine being scared of the dark and worrying that there are monsters under your bed (misinterpretation of threat). The trigger is bedtime and turning the light off for sleep. When you start panicking and feeling anxious, you decide to turn the light on. You may go to sleep with the light on, try to stay awake, arrange to have someone check under your bed before sleep, or request that someone sits on guard at the foot of your bed (possibly teddy or another equally brave toy). This immediately makes you feel better and in your mind it significantly reduces the threat of a monster crawling out from under your bed and attacking you at night (as we all know monsters are scared of light and will only pounce if you are blissfully unconscious in sleep!). Over time you become dependent on these defences and can no longer go to sleep without teddy or without the light off, despite the fact there were no monsters present in the first place! It is a vicious cycle that now continues to spin, even though the perceived threat was non-existent.

I am not trying to trivialise anxiety and obsessional disorders with this example, as I know how distressing they can be for all involved. I just wanted to illustrate how behavioural responses can become part of the problem if left unchecked.

How you are part of the problem

GIVING REASSURANCE

As we have already discussed, seeking reassurance is a type of
safety behaviour and it can take many forms. Reassurance can
be sought in different ways, including via direct or round-about
questions, watching TV, reading the news, and visiting medical
professionals. It can be very obvious in some cases when people
are seeking reassurance from you – and in some cases it can
be very tricky to know. I have worked for years in the field of
anxiety and obsessional problems and I can still be caught out by
someone who is cleverly seeking reassurance in some way!

Don't get me wrong; giving reassurance to someone you love
is a very normal and natural thing to do. We give reassurance all
the time in our relationships with others: 'That outfit looks fine';
'Being five minutes late is okay'; 'You haven't put on weight'. So
you will know that even if you give reassurance, it doesn't mean
it is true or that the person believes it. If your partner has put on
a small amount of weight and asks you, 'Have I put on weight?',
the truth is they know the answer already. And if you say 'no' they
will not believe you, or if you say 'yes', they will be upset anyway.
It is a lose-lose situation. In the context of anxiety or obsessional
problems, it is the same thing – it doesn't matter what you say.
Your loved one will still be anxious and doubt whether you are
telling the truth, and then will want more and more reassurance.

Think about whether you are asked for reassurance by your
loved one in relation to their anxiety problem. It can be hard to
separate "normal" reassurance that would be appropriate in any
situation and "unhelpful" reassurance in the case of anxiety and
obsessional problems. If you are unsure, I would err on the side
of caution and treat any requests for reassurance as ones that
are safety behaviours. When I am in clinic, I ask the families and
partners of my clients to stop giving reassurance. I say this in front
of my clients so they know that it is happening and to expect it,
and that it is part of the treatment process.

I suggest that you tell your loved one that you understand that giving reassurance is not actually helping them face their problems and that you are going to stop giving reassurance when they request it. Be clear that you love them, and that this is not as a punishment, but that you do not want to do anything that contributes to the ongoing nature of their problem, for example:

'I love you very much and want you to get better. I now know that when you ask for reassurance it is to try to reduce your anxiety, but it doesn't work long term. Seeking reassurance is unhelpful and can keep this problem going, and I don't want to be part of that. If you seek reassurance from me, I am going to remind you that I will not give it, but that I care about you very much and want to find other ways to help you overcome this problem.'

You may have to be prepared for some arguments with your loved one. In the throes of anxiety, they will not be reasonable and may demand reassurance from you, especially if they used to get it from you previously. But hold your ground and eventually they will learn that you will not give them the reassurance. And don't be too hard on yourself if you occasionally get tricked into giving it either – I still get caught out despite my many years of practice. It can be helpful to share your new "not giving reassurance" approach with other family members too so you can have some support and ensure that you are all being consistent and someone else doesn't become the "go to" person for reassurance.

FACILITATING AVOIDANCE

Another way to get caught out is by helping your loved one avoid things that they are worried about or believe will trigger an anxiety response. Again, this is a very normal thing to do for people we love. If they really dislike something or it causes them agitation, we try to help them avoid it.

It could be that you are avoiding things that you enjoy or want to do because of your loved one's problem, or you are helping them avoid certain things. Commonly people make excuses for their loved one's unwillingness to attend events. So, from this point, please stop making excuses for your loved one's anxiety problem – it is not your loved one you are helping, but their problem. And if you are avoiding doing things that you want to do, stop this. It is not helping your loved one, and you are missing out too. It is better for you to go solo to events and get some enjoyment out of them. Again, it is best to explain your reasons for doing this to your loved one, so they are aware that they can no longer depend on your excuses.

TAKING PART IN RITUALS OR SAFETY BEHAVIOURS

In the case of the obsessive compulsive disorders, you may be asked to take part in some of your loved one's rituals or compulsions. I have seen family members help with cleaning and checking rituals, partners hiding knives and other objects of concern, family members showering and washing more, partners helping their loved one retrace their steps, and so on. Often family members can't quite recall how they got involved in the rituals and seem a bit surprised when they find out they are taking part in them. It can creep up on you when you start it little by little. It will be no surprise here when I tell you to STOP it. For all the same reasons outlined above, you are only helping facilitate the problem and keep it spinning in its vicious cycle. Explain to your loved one that you are stopping partaking in rituals as you know it is unhelpful and only giving the OCD more room to grow.

Tips on changing the way you respond:

- Communicate your plans
- Be clear why you are changing your behaviour
- Explain that it is to help them, not hurt them

- Ensure a consistent approach with other family members and friends
- Expect some conflict
- Stand your ground – it will get easier over time

WHAT IF MY LOVED ONE'S ANXIETY PROBLEM GETS WORSE ONCE I CHANGE MY RESPONSES?

This might well happen. By taking away access to safety behaviours, your loved one may seem to get worse. But believe me, you did not cause the problem and the anxiety will get worse anyway without good treatment. You are just taking away one of the supports that is propping up the problem. Your loved one might have to feel the full extent of their problem before they will acknowledge it *is* a problem and seek help.

I have also seen new safety behaviours develop and take the place of ones that have become less effective or are now unavailable. Again, don't worry if this happens – it would have happened eventually. And even if there are new safety behaviours, it frees you from a burden if they are no longer dependent on you.

CHAPTER SUMMARY

- There is a **vicious cycle** present in anxiety and obsessional problems in which the behavioural responses keep the problem going.
- Your behaviour, usually unintentionally, can contribute to this vicious cycle.
- The most common ways are through giving reassurance, facilitating avoidance and partaking in rituals.

- It is normal to want to reduce your loved one's suffering but by stopping these responses, you can stop giving the problem space to grow.
- You should communicate your plans to change your responses clearly and be consistent in your approach.
- It is possible that the anxiety problem will get worse or your loved one develops a new safety behaviour if you change your behaviour, but it is not your fault and would likely have happened anyway. Sometimes people need to experience the full extent of their problem before acknowledging they need help to overcome it.

CHAPTER SIX

CURRENT TREATMENTS FOR ANXIETY AND OBSESSIONAL DISORDERS

I'm sure you have searched the internet and spoken to other people – possibly mental health professionals – to find treatments that actually work for your loved one's anxiety or obsessional problem. It can be a bit of a minefield to sort through the information (and misinformation) that you receive. In this chapter I present treatments that have a body of research behind them proving that they work directly on the mental health problem.

Of course, eating well, sleeping better, getting exercise, de-stressing and being more mindful is beneficial for mental health in general, and we can all do more of this! But they do not solve an anxiety or obsessional problem on their own. Your loved one will need an active treatment – either a psychological therapy, a medication, or perhaps both.

Accessing Therapy

The intensity and type of intervention will depend on several factors: accessibility, affordability, and the severity of the problem.

ACCESSIBILITY
This refers to how easy it is to access good treatment. You may live in a remote area or in a place that does not provide the

recommended mental health treatments. You may only be able to access group therapy rather than individual therapy. The good news is that most treatments can be self-administered for the less severe problems and the internet age has opened up more options for therapy. I have successfully provided remote therapy over the phone and online, and many therapists now offer this an option.

AFFORDABILITY

Like most things in life, good treatment will cost money. However, this is one of those situations where it is much better paying for good quality treatment if you can afford it, as it should work and will save you from greater cost in the future – particularly if the problem becomes worse and causes more missed work days, difficulty working, and more associated costs such as childcare and transport. I know it is expensive; not everyone can afford private individual therapy. But there are also very good inexpensive (or free!) options such as self-help books, computer-based therapy, and group therapy, all of which are effective forms of treatment. Private health insurance will often fund therapy or part of the cost. In the UK we have the wonderful NHS which provides "free" treatment (of course, it is not actually "free" as it is funded by taxpayers). There is the issue of it being under-resourced with long waiting lists, but it is still a very good option if cost is an issue.

SEVERITY OF THE PROBLEM

Treatments and their effectiveness will of course depend on how severe the problem is. For anxiety and obsessional problems in the "mild to moderate" severity range, most can be treated by self-help books or programmes, computerised treatment, group therapy or individual treatment. For people with "moderate" problems, therapy and medication are recommended. Medication may be used as a treatment, but people can still get better without medication if they have the right therapy. Medication is more important when people suffer severe anxiety and obsessional problems, and in these cases, it is recommended to be taken alongside psychological treatments.

How do you determine how severe a problem is? Well, professionals use clinical tools (questionnaires), their own assessments, and a good dose of common sense. For example, if you have OCD but live a relatively normal life and it doesn't bother you too much, then you would be considered a "mild" case. But if you have OCD and are housebound and dependent on other people to care for you, spending most of your day caught up in rituals, then you would be considered "severe".

There is a category that includes "treatment resistant" problems, which means the problem is severe and longstanding and the recommended treatments have not worked to date. Treatment resistant cases are very rare, and even in this group of people I have seen successful results with medication combined with intensive treatments. If you are unsure about the severity of your problem, I would suggest seeking an opinion from your doctor, psychologist or other mental health professional.

Cognitive Behavioural Therapy (CBT)

This is by far the best and most effective therapy – it is supported by years of research and clinical trials and we know it works. Many people come to my clinic saying they have tried hypnotherapy, massage, acupuncture, generic counselling, and other holistic treatments but that they have not worked. That is because there is no evidence that they work in the case of anxiety and obsessional problems. They might help people feel better in the short term and improve wellbeing in other ways, but they do not effectively treat anxiety or obsessional disorders.

CBT is the study of the relationships between things that happen in your life, how you interpret them, and your physiological, emotional and behavioural responses to them. What we describe as "cognition" is the way you think, what you believe, and how you interpret things. The "physiological" is your bodily reaction, the "emotional" is your feeling response, and the "behavioural" is what you do about it, physically or mentally. CBT is designed to interrupt the vicious cycle of the anxiety or obsessional problems that I discussed in the previous chapter. It is evidence-based and it hands over the tools of treatment, recovery and maintenance of that recovery to the individual – so the therapists are *not* the secret holders of information! The knowledge is meant to be shared and this is why there are so many free or easily accessible versions of CBT available.

CBT can be delivered effectively in individual therapy sessions (in person or remotely), in group therapy led by a trained CBT professional, via online CBT programmes (called Computerised Cognitive Behavioural Therapy or CCBT), by self-help books and by telephone.[xv] CBT requires the person to proactively and actively engage with the treatment and there are homework tasks set between sessions.

COMPONENTS OF CBT

If we go back to our vicious cycle, we will see that CBT attempts to change the "interpretation" part (the cognitions) and modify the behavioural responses.

COGNITIVE RESTRUCTURING/THOUGHT CHALLENGING

Using various strategies, CBT shows you how to change your thoughts. In the case of anxiety and obsessional problems, it shows you how to change your "misinterpretation" of a threat and the overestimated likelihood of the feared outcome. For example, someone who worries about having a panic attack and "going crazy" due to the panic would, in CBT, be presented with information about anxiety and panic attacks and be shown the evidence both for and against the case that they may "go crazy". This is so they can correctly evaluate the likelihood of it happening.

Once they realise it is very unlikely they'll "go crazy", they are able to change their belief or "misinterpretation of threat". For example, they may now think, *I feel overwhelmed by the anxiety and it feels like something awful will happen, but I know this is the anxiety in my body and it will pass.*

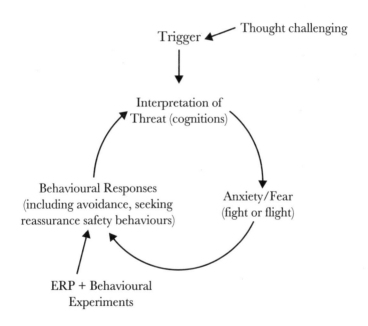

EXPOSURE RESPONSE PREVENTION (ERP)

This component of CBT is used for the treatment of OCD and BDD, but it can also be used in other anxiety problems if indicated. It refers to exposing the individual to the thoughts, images, objects and situations that make them anxious and trigger their obsessions, then preventing the unhelpful responses that follow (ritual or compulsions). For example, if someone with OCD is worried about contamination and excessively washes their hands, then ERP would likely involve touching something they consider "dirty" and then touching their clothes or hair (door handles and taps are a good starting point). They would do this without wearing gloves, washing their hands afterwards or using some other perceived hygienic practice.

BEHAVIOURAL EXPERIMENTS

This is a way for people to challenge their unhelpful behavioural responses by setting experiments to test out predictions. This helps by changing the thinking too – in particular the perceived fearful outcome. For example, someone with social anxiety disorder might set an experiment to test out his belief that everyone will laugh at him during a work meeting, and his experiment would be to speak up at the meeting (as opposed to avoid it) and see what happens.

APPLIED RELAXATION (AR)

This is a technique used in the treatment of GAD, which teaches the individual how to systematically relax their body reasonably quickly and overcome the physiological symptoms of anxiety. It usually involves Progressive Muscle Relaxation (PMR) in which different parts of the body are tensed then relaxed in turn. I discuss AR in more detail in Part Two, Chapter Five.

SELF-GUIDED VS GUIDED SELF-HELP

Your loved one may undertake treatment via self-help methods. This means that they are learning CBT and applying it on their own, usually with a CBT book or online CBT programme. This is known as "self-guided" help. If there is some professional support involved this would be "guided self-help". Professional support in this case would only be brief phone support, text messaging or online chats in self-help programmes. The support is usually minimal and is not meant to replicate individual therapy sessions with a professional.

PSYCHOEDUCATION

This refers to receiving accurate information about mental health conditions and it is often delivered in groups, possibly run by a hospital, charity, support group or a mental health clinic. It is general information and not individualised for each person.

FREQUENCY AND INTENSITY

Whilst most CBT programmes recommend that sessions are delivered weekly, this is general advice for mild to moderate disorders. There is emerging evidence that intensive treatments – as in longer and possibly more frequent sessions – are appropriate for treating moderate to severe anxiety problems. Certainly when working with moderate to severe OCD clients I have seen that having more sessions per week can be a very effective treatment format.

There is proof that single-session treatments for some phobias are successful forms of treatment. I have also worked with several clients who have been successfully treated for panic disorder in under five sessions. So, whilst it is important to have sessions close enough together to ensure the best outcome of therapy, the number of sessions can vary depending on each client. Also, if people are making good progress, then I will often spread out the final sessions over longer periods, perhaps once a month for review and follow up.

Medication

Medication can be very helpful for some people and give them the support and boost they need to undertake CBT, but not everyone needs medication. Often it allows them to engage in treatment and helps stabilise their mood in order to get the best out of treatment.

On the other hand, I have also seen many people get better without taking medication. Current advice states that if someone has mild to moderate anxiety or obsessional problems, they do not necessarily need medication to get better. A good course of CBT is an effective treatment on its own. However, some people might have co-morbid depression and require medication for their mood. If they have a more severe anxiety or obsessional problem, the evidence is that medication can help alongside a good course of treatment. There is no right or wrong answer here, and it will depend on individual preference as well as the advice from a psychologist or medical doctor.

If your loved one is currently taking a medication or considering one, then they should speak to their doctor, who will give them the information they need and prescribe the medication. I have provided a brief overview of the types of medication that will likely be considered, but this review does not replace the need for individualised medical advice.

Please note, though, that the actual names of the medication will change depending which country you are in, as different drug companies will produce them. Which medication is prescribed will depend on individual factors such as medication history and medical background, and the prescribed doses will vary within a recommended range. Sometimes doctors may even combine medications (called augmentation) for people if it is clinically indicated (usually in the case of severe obsessional problems).

ANTIDEPRESSANTS

These are frequently prescribed for anxiety and obsessional problems and can help if your loved one is also suffering from depression. They are a non-addictive medication and safe if taken as prescribed.

SELECTIVE SEROTONIN REUPTAKE INHIBITORS (SSRIS)

SSRIS are a common medication for anxiety and obsessional problems. They are part of a family of antidepressants that have been proven to be effective for anxiety, OCD and depression.

SEROTONIN NOREPINEPHRINE REUPTAKE INHIBITORS (SNRIS)

SNRIS are another group of antidepressants and have shown clinical effectiveness in the treatment of anxiety.

TRICYCLIC ANTIDEPRESSANTS (TCAS)

In some cases, a tricyclic antidepressant may be prescribed. These are less common and usually only prescribed if SSRI's or SNRI's are not working or are not indicated for other medical reasons.

MONOAMINE OXIDASE INHIBITORS (MAOIS)

MAOIs are one of the first types of antidepressant developed. They are effective, but usually newer antidepressants such as SSRI or SNRI's are now used as they are considered less restrictive and have fewer side effects. MAOIs typically require diet restrictions and avoiding certain other medications, as they can cause high blood pressure when taken with certain foods or medications. Despite this, these medications are still a good option when other medications cannot be prescribed.

ANXIETY-SPECIFIC MEDICATIONS

BETA BLOCKERS

Beta blockers are a medication that can be used to manage the physical symptoms of anxiety. They are not addictive and can be used in specific situations under the clear advice of a doctor.

BENZODIAZEPINES

Benzodiazepines are anti-anxiety medications that can be prescribed in emergency situations to provide immediate relief. However, they are not recommended for long-term management of an anxiety problem because they *are* addictive and can continue to mask physiological symptoms, enabling those taking such medication to believe they don't need psychological treatment. The use of benzodiazepines can then become a safety behaviour which, as we now know, is not helpful.

All medications come with a long list of potential side effects, but not everyone will get the same side-effects as every person responds differently to them.

Here is a summary of the current recommended treatments for anxiety and obsessional problems at the time of publication:[xvi]

> **Medication will not solve an anxiety or obsessional problem alone – it should be combined with good quality CBT.**

DISORDER	MILD	MODERATE	SEVERE
Generalised anxiety disorder	• Individual self-guided self-help • Individual guided self-help CBT • Psychoeducational group based on CBT	• CBT or Applied Relaxation Therapy • Medication (SSRI – sertraline). If SSRI is ineffective, offer SNRI. If unresponsive to SNRI, offer a TCA	• Medication and intensive psychological treatment
Panic disorder (with or without agoraphobia)	• Individual self-guided self-help • Individual guided self-help CBT • Psychoeducational group based on CBT	• CBT • Medication if the disorder is long-standing or the individual has not benefited from psychological treatment – an SSRI or TCA	• CBT including home-based treatment if attendance at clinic is difficult • Medication
Obsessive compulsive disorder	• Self-guided self-help CBT • Exposure and Response Prevention (ERP) using self-help materials and/or telephone support • Group CBT including ERP	• CBT and ERP with a trained therapist • Medication (SSRI)	• Combined treatment of therapy (CBT & ERP) and medication (SSRI)
Body dysmorphic disorder	• Group or individual CBT including ERP	• Individual CBT including ERP, and Medication (SSRI)	• Combined treatment of intensive therapy (CBT ERP) and medication (SSRI)

Continued

DISORDER	MILD	MODERATE	SEVERE
Social anxiety disorder	• Individual CBT	• Individual CBT • SSRI or, if unresponsive, an SNRI. If unresponsive to the SNRI, an MAOI • If the person declines CBT, offer short-term psychodynamic psychotherapy specifically developed to treat social anxiety[xvii]	• Combined treatment of Individual CBT and SSRI or, if unresponsive, an SNRI. If unresponsive to the SNRI, an MAOI
Illness anxiety disorder[xviii]	• Self-guided internet CBT[xix]	• Individual CBT possibly combined with antidepressant medication (SSRI)	
Phobias	• Self-guided CBT including exposure therapy	• Individual CBT involving exposure therapy	• May require intensive treatment

In the case of people who are severely unwell and unable to live without considerable help, hospitalisation is always an option. It may be that they are hospitalised against their wishes in line with mental health legislation, or they may opt to stay at the hospital voluntarily. However, whilst they are in hospital, they would most likely receive both medication and CBT treatment.

What happens if treatment doesn't work?

There are many reasons why treatments might not work. It could be that the type of treatment was not matched properly to your loved one's needs, that the sessions were too far apart (standard weekly CBT sessions are recommended for most anxiety or obsessional problems), that it was not CBT, or the therapist was not trained specifically in CBT for anxiety or obsessions. It may be that your loved one was too depressed to engage in treatment, isn't motivated to change, or that the full extent of the anxiety problem was being disguised by safety behaviours (another reason to stop your role in them!).

These are only a few possible reasons. But do remain hopeful, as this means that the right treatment SHOULD work. I have lost count of the people I have treated who reported unsuccessful treatments previously for their anxiety or obsessional problem. The most common reasons were that they either tried a medication without CBT or that the "CBT" was *not actually* CBT or the *right type* of CBT. Many people may say they are trained in CBT but are either not trained properly or have not had enough training or experience. But rest assured, most of these people got better with the right CBT. Even in the case of medication, if one particular drug doesn't work for your loved one, another might, so don't worry if your loved one hasn't responded to the first medication tried.

How can we find a therapist trained in CBT for anxiety and obsessional problems?

In most places there should be a centralised register of people who are competently trained in CBT. In the UK it is the British Association of Behavioural and Cognitive Psychotherapists (BABCP), or the British Psychological Society (BPS). If where you live does not have a professional CBT organisation, I would recommend trying the National Psychologist Association. Psychologists are required by law to have a high level of training, ongoing professional training and supervision, and are usually well qualified in CBT. This professional body will also be able to tell you if there are other regulated organisations that provide CBT.

If you find a therapist who claims to be qualified in CBT, do not be afraid to ask for evidence of their qualifications, training and experience in treating anxiety and obsessional problems. If you were getting a tradesman to install a new kitchen in your house you would ask about his experience, see photos of his previous work, and possibly read some reviews from other clients. Your loved one's mental health is no different, and it is a big commitment to make. If your loved one is too unwell, unsure or anxious to do it themselves, then ask them if it is okay if you ask these questions. You may also consider doing your own research on good therapists locally or available online, through forums, mental health charities, or via your friends and family network.

Remember, one in three people suffer from anxiety at some time in their life, so it is very likely that people you know will be able to recommend a good therapist.

Another tip would be for you and your loved one to read a self-help CBT book on anxiety and/or obsessional problems. Then you can check if the therapy is following a similar course to what is recommended in the book. At any time, if you or your loved one is not sure on whether it is the right type of treatment, they should speak to their therapist. It might well be that they are following protocol but it was not clearly communicated, or your loved one was too anxious to take the information on board. I always encourage my clients to ask me questions and query my methods in order to properly understand the therapy and as a check for me to make sure I'm following the right path in treatment. I also always offer my clients the option to audio-record the sessions and take them home to listen to them later. Not all clients like this idea, but given that some of them are so anxious in sessions and may not be able to pay attention to all the information, I want to make sure they have the opportunity to listen to it again.

What can I expect during my loved one's treatment?

CONFIDENTIALITY

First, even though you are very involved in your loved one's life, it does not mean you will be very involved in their therapy sessions. Therapy and medical appointments are confidential, and we are not allowed to break confidentiality and tell you anything. This is often very hard when I know partners and family are desperate to help their loved one, but unless your loved one consents to sharing the information, we cannot speak to you about the therapy, including prognosis or treatment recommendations. The only times we can share information with you without your loved one's consent is if we are worried about their safety – for example if they disclose suicidal thoughts – or the safety of someone close to you – for example if children are suffering neglect due to their illness.

Your loved one can consent to sharing information with you. I always discuss with my clients what they would like to share with their family and partners and we arrange joint sessions in which we can discuss the problem and the recommended treatment plan. This is also very useful when you are partaking in safety behaviours and facilitating the problem.

I believe it is very important to involve family and partners in the treatment. I should say that most people are happy to share information with their loved ones and feel supported when they want to join in the therapy. If your loved one does not want to share information with you, it may be because they are embarrassed or ashamed or they find it too overwhelming. They may choose to share only part of the therapy information with you and not want you to listen to the recordings, which is fine. People are vulnerable in therapy sessions and often disclose information that is incredibly sensitive and personal, and you should respect that. It is okay and appropriate for them to have an "inside world" that is just for them.

BEING A CO-THERAPIST

In certain situations, it may be helpful for you to take on the role of "co-therapist". This is so you can help your loved one undertake parts of their CBT treatment at home. I often enlist the help of family and partners to undertake some of the challenging experiments in CBT, which I discuss later in Part Two, Chapter Four. If your loved one is open to this idea, then it can be useful to plan experiments together alongside therapy, either with a therapist's help or – if your loved one is doing self-guided CBT or an online programme – you may choose the experiments together.

This can be a very satisfying role, although you must remember to be patient and compassionate as your loved one will find these exposure experiments challenging. You will be asking them to face something that they are very scared of – even if you think it is something silly. When faced with exposure tasks that they find challenging, so many of my clients with OCD say, 'I wish I had that handwashing OCD, because it is so silly that it wouldn't be a problem to stop washing my hands.' Yet this is exactly why they don't have handwashing OCD – because it doesn't frighten them!

UPS AND DOWNS IN THE PATH OF TREATMENT AND RECOVERY

The path of treatment and recovery never runs smoothly. Having treatment and recovering from an anxiety or obsessional problem is like recovering from any illness – there will be ups and downs before a stable recovery position is made. It may be difficult to know if your loved one is making progress but there can be small steps that you may not see immediately, and there will definitely be days when it seems like they might be taking a step backwards. But as progress is made, these days will become fewer and further apart.

In fact, if someone didn't have up and down days during treatment with me, I would be concerned. Anxiety and obsessional problems are emotional problems and there will be emotional consequences. I sometimes call these "emotional hangovers" which is when someone feels flat or more anxious following therapy sessions or intense exposure treatments. There will be peaks and troughs along the journey, but what matters is that the general trend is in the right direction.

Because CBT is designed to hand over the tools of treatment to the client, we would also expect people to continue to improve even when treatment sessions have finished. My goal is to discharge people when they are 75% recovered, and they can continue to make the remainder 25% improvement on their own. They know what to do and how to do it, so there is no reason they won't continue to get better.

CHAPTER SUMMARY

- There are effective treatments for anxiety and obsessional problems.
- CBT is the best talking therapy and is available in many formats, including individual therapy sessions, group therapy, online treatment programmes, remote therapy with a therapist, and self-help books.
- Medication combined with CBT is the recommended treatment for moderate to severe anxiety problems.

- The type of treatment will depend on accessibility, affordability and severity of the problem.
- There are many reasons why treatment might not have worked in the past, but this should not stop your loved one having treatment again and recovering from their problem.
- Confidentiality means you will not know what is said in your loved one's therapy session, and therapists and doctors cannot provide you with any information without your loved one's consent.
- It can be very helpful to have partners and family members involved in the treatment process.
- Like any illness or injury, the journey to recovery is bumpy, marked by good days and bad. This is normal and to be expected during treatment for an anxiety or obsessional problem.

PART TWO

TIME FOR ACTION

CHAPTER ONE
UNDERSTAND YOUR RESPONSIBILITIES
AND DEFINE YOUR ROLES

I have already mentioned this earlier in the book, but it is such an important sentiment that I am going to dedicate a whole section to it to drive home the message. Despite what you may be telling yourself, YOU ARE NOT RESPONSIBLE FOR MAKING YOUR LOVED ONE BETTER.

You cannot be responsible because you cannot change how someone acts. This is a fact, albeit a bit of an annoying one at times. Therefore you cannot be responsible for them making the necessary changes to get better. It does not stop you wanting to help your loved one get better and feeling frustrated when they don't engage in treatment, or when they won't acknowledge they have a problem.

I am not saying give up on them or stop caring, as this would be very harsh and impossible to do anyway. But you *can* take a step back, think about how you are responding to their anxiety or obsessional problem, and remove the demands you are placing on yourself to make them better. A positive outcome will be that you may feel less frustrated and annoyed at your loved one and less stressed overall.

Think about it – when things are your responsibility, it is much harder to relax knowing that people are depending on you, whether this is at work or home. Washing your child's team bibs for sport, making cakes or setting up a stall for a school fête, volunteering to pick up shopping for someone, making sure a deadline is met at work, getting to appointments on time… when things are your responsibility and you have more control over them, then you feel more pressured and frustrated if you don't live up to the demands. However, if things are out of your control, then you don't feel as worried about them. Instead of getting to work on time during a snowstorm, it becomes much less stressful if the public transport systems have shut down and there is physically no way to get to work (which happens in London at least once a year!).

For example, it may be stressful if you have a work deadline and the whole team needs to work towards it, but Jack from IT is not able to help because he is off very sick with the flu. It is outside your control and you will deal with it somehow. This is the same for anxiety and obsessional problems – you cannot control the illness, nor can you control your loved one's behaviour, including their desire and motivation to get better. If your loved one had broken their leg in a bike accident on the way to work, you wouldn't hold yourself responsible for the accident or their recovery. If your loved one had high blood pressure, you wouldn't hold yourself responsible for making sure they took their medication and made all the lifestyle changes the doctor recommended. Sure, you would support them and make the changes easier – for example, serving up healthier meals and exercising alongside them – but you cannot force them to do the right thing. It is no different in the case of anxiety or obsessional problems. You cannot force people to make changes; you can only make it easier for them to make the changes.

It's not your responsibility

The reality is – and sometimes this is difficult to hear – that assuming responsibility for their illness and recovery is actually preventing your loved one from being a self-realised, problem solving, responsible adult. You are not helping someone by trying to force them to get help – they will end up blaming you and resenting you for forcing them to have treatment and for the lack of progress they make.

It may be that your loved one is not ready to acknowledge their problem or even the extent of it. It may be that you are trying to force them to get help while at the same time partaking in safety behaviours which camouflage the full extent of the problem. It may be that your loved one's problem has to deteriorate before they admit to having a problem or realise the impact of it, but this will have to happen anyway. You taking responsibility for their problem and treatment will only delay this from happening.

There is also evidence that people who are motivated before engaging in CBT treatment do better in treatment and maintain the treatment gains for longer.[xx] So that is even more reason to allow your loved one to come to their own conclusion that they need to get some help.

If you feel overly responsible for your loved one's problem and for getting them better, perhaps you are engaging in a few thinking problems of your own (see Part One, Chapter Three), most likely "magnified duty" – believing you are overly responsible for your loved one's health and discounting the fact that they are responsible for their own behaviour – and/or "perceived control" – thinking that you have more control over their behaviour than you do. You may also be placing demands on yourself by thinking you "should" or "must" get your loved one better and by seeking guarantees about the future that your loved one will get better.

See, it's very easy to fall into unhelpful thinking patterns! If you identify with any of these, then you will need to come up with a more helpful way of thinking. This is exactly what we do in CBT treatment – take unhelpful beliefs, identify any thinking problems, challenge them with facts (as I have done in the preceding paragraphs) and come up with more accurate, helpful ways of thinking. I have made some suggestions below, but you may come up with your own new approaches that allow you to step back from taking responsibility for your loved one's problem.

UNHELPFUL THOUGHTS	NEW HELPFUL THOUGHTS
I am responsible for making my loved one better.	I cannot be responsible for anyone else's behaviour, despite wanting the best outcome for them.
I should reduce their distress and anxiety.	By trying to reduce their anxiety, I am helping them hide from the full extent of their problem and letting the problem continue.
If I don't help reduce their anxiety or try to get them treatment, it means I don't love them.	I love them so much that it makes sense I want to reduce their suffering, but in reality, I am not helping and could be making the problem worse.
If I don't try to force them to get help, they will get worse and it will be my fault.	I cannot make them engage in treatment, and if they get worse it will not be my fault. In fact, they may have to get worse before they can start to get better.
If I don't take responsibility to get them better, they won't take responsibility to get better themselves.	I want them to become a self-realised responsible adult, so I need to give them the opportunity to get better and grow.

COMPASSIONATE HELP

Just to be clear, I am not saying don't help your loved one. I just want you to be fair to yourself and be realistic about what you are able to achieve. You can help and support them in a compassionate way, within limits. The key words here are "compassion" and "limits".

COMPASSION

Compassion is defined as a *"strong feeling of sympathy and sadness for the suffering or bad luck of others and a wish to help them."*[xxi]

What this means is that you can sympathise with your loved one and the distress and anxiety they feel. You can care for them and help them in a non-judgemental and non-critical way.

Compassion does not mean trying to solve the problem for them or pointing out the irrationality of their ways. For example, if your loved one is feeling anxious about an upcoming event, you can sympathise with them but encourage them to face their fear at the same time.

LIMITS

Limits refers to the help you can provide that is within your capability and that is not continuing to keep the vicious cycle spinning. By not facilitating avoidance, giving reassurance or playing into safety behaviours, you are in fact helping your loved one – even if at times it feels like you are not because they are anxious and distressed.

Jonah and Susie *have a twenty-four-year-old daughter, Ivy, who is suffering from severe OCD around causing harm to others, particularly children. The impact of her OCD is profound and she is often distressed about leaving the house. Susie and Jonah would regularly stay at home instead of going out in order to reassure Ivy, provide her company, and run all of her errands.*

However, after speaking to a CBT therapist on the best way forward, they have now decided to stop facilitating her avoidance along with re-starting the activities they used to enjoy – going to the cinema, visiting friends and hosting barbeques. They will only buy essential groceries and will not be buying Ivy clothes and make-up when they go shopping. They will also not provide OCD reassurance. Susie has researched some good local CBT therapists and has offered to help pay for treatment sessions and drive Ivy to appointments. Whilst they expect Ivy to be more anxious in the short term, they hope this will enable her to take the first steps towards having treatment.

Define your role

Now it is time to consider what steps you can take to help your loved one and make a plan with them about getting better. If your loved one is not committed to getting better, you should still make a plan for yourself about what you are prepared to do – or not do – in the case of assisting with safety behaviours. If your loved one is motivated to participate in treatment, that's great news! And it means that you will need to define your role in the process and manage your loved one's expectations. I suggest talking to your loved one as you work through the following chapters, as an agreed plan will be much easier to implement. If your loved one does not want to discuss this or the conversation ends in an argument, you might find the chapter on communication and conflict useful as you will still need to communicate what you are planning to change.

Defining your role either during treatment or in the case that your loved one does not want to get help will help focus your energy on the roles that you can and want to do. These are all roles that families and partners I have worked with have taken on, and the list is just a guide – you may have other roles that I have not included. Keeping in mind that you can wear multiple hats at once and the roles can overlap, you may choose to be a Supporter and Financier, or you may be a Co-Therapist, Friend and Cheerleader. I have not included the roles of Partner and Family Member because you are doing these anyway (and they may be less optional!):

- **Supporter** – support your loved one whenever they need support, whatever that looks like.
- **Co-therapist** – take an active role in treatment and be part of the exposure tasks and experiments.
- **Advocate** – learn about the pathways to good treatment and fight for your loved one's access to good treatment.
- **Friend** – be there for the ups and downs, laugh and cry together, and listen without judgement.

- **Financier** – fund the cost of therapy, transport to and from sessions, cover the rent or mortgage bills, etc., if your loved one can't work whilst having treatment.
- **Cheerleader** – positively cheer on your loved one for all their achievements.
- **Realist** – understand it is a hard road for your loved one and that ups and downs are the reality of treatment.
- **Humourist** – because sometimes laughter is just what you need.
- **Believer** – retain hope and believe your loved one can make positive changes.
- **Human** – this is to remind yourself that you are human too, and that therefore you are vulnerable to the human emotions of annoyance, frustration and anger. Understand that you will also have your ups and downs during this process.

HOW CAN I BE A CO-THERAPIST?

One of the more formalised roles is that of co-therapist. You may take on this role where it is difficult for your loved one to make it to therapy sessions and you need to lead them through the exposure and experiment tasks, or if your loved one is doing self-guided treatment and asks for your help along the way. It is an excellent way to support your loved one and help them during the treatment. It would usually involve helping your loved one undertake the active parts of treatment, exposure and response prevention, and behavioural experiments. I will talk about these more in Part Two, Chapter Four.

As a co-therapist, it is important to remain positive and encouraging yet firm. And you should do everything that your loved one is expected to do. For example, if you ask your loved one to not do their hair or wear make-up one day to the shops (to treat their BDD), then you should not do this either. Or if you ask your loved one to pet a dog in the case of dog phobia, then you should also pet the dog. As a co-therapist it is important to know when to switch off from this role too – your loved one might appreciate your encouragement during the exposure tasks but not when they are watching their favourite TV show that evening! Believe me (or believe my husband) – no one wants a therapist around *all* the time.

PRACTICAL SUPPORT

Another thing to consider is the practical elements of support. There are many ways you may be able to help someone who needs treatment for an anxiety or obsessional problem. These include helping your loved one find a CBT therapist or some self-help books, babysitting if they need to go to appointments, or if they are doing the sessions online and have no childcare (obviously if you are co-parents you would just "parent" your own children), offering to drop them at appointments and wait for them, or cooking them meals if they get home late from treatment sessions or are spending the evening doing self-help sessions.

CHAPTER SUMMARY

- It is not your responsibility to make your loved one better. Only your loved one can change their behaviour, although you can support them in a compassionate way.
- If you feel overly responsible towards your loved one, you may have some thinking problems of your own which you need to challenge and you will need to come up with new, more helpful ways of thinking.

- By allowing your loved one to take responsibility for their problem, you are giving them the opportunity to develop and grow as a person.
- If someone is motivated to address their anxiety or obsessional problem, they are more likely to make progress in treatment and maintain treatment gains.
- It is helpful to define your role for yourself and your loved one to manage everyone's expectations.
- Offering practical support is incredibly valuable when people are undertaking treatment.

CHAPTER TWO
HAVE THE CONVERSATION: CONFLICT AND COMMUNICATION

I have no doubt that you have experienced conflict in relation to your loved one's anxiety or obsessional problem. It might be conflict with your loved one, or another family member, on how to deal with your loved one's problem. It might be with professionals involved in your loved one's care, or friends and others affected by your loved one's problem. Primarily this chapter is written with the conflicts you have directly with your loved one – about or because of their anxiety or obsessional problem – in mind. But there is no reason the strategies should not be used in the other examples.

Also, this chapter is not about avoiding conflict, because conflict will happen when people have different ideas about how things should work. But the way you approach these potentially conflicting situations and the way you communicate with others can make the disagreements feel less personal and less hurtful. It can also hopefully allow you to take on board what the other person is saying. Remember, in arguments, each person has a valid point of view – the goal is not forcing an agreed viewpoint, but providing a way that you can move forward from disagreement.

Conversations can be difficult

Conversations can be difficult and emotionally fraught, but this is no reason to avoid them. Dialogues are needed for positive change in the future and without them, nothing will change and dysfunctional patterns will continue. Avoiding conversations that you need to have also allows emotions like resentment and anger to fester. Conversations that are hard to have are often the most important, so do not avoid them.

EXPECTATIONS

It is helpful to have realistic expectations about difficult conversations. Often conflict happens when we try to win someone over to our own point of view, but this doesn't really make sense as we are all individuals with different experiences in life, different values and different goals. So do not expect conversations to resolve perfectly, or even to resolve at all. You may not feel better at the end of the conversation, but this is not the purpose. The point of having difficult conversations is to allow things to be said, having your feelings heard and allowing your loved one's thoughts and feelings to be heard too. It is about opening up dialogues rather than solving issues in that moment.

Often we expect things to resolve quickly if we decide to have a "serious talk" with somebody, but that's unfair on them and unrealistic, particularly if it's the first time they are hearing what you are saying or if what you are saying is difficult for them to hear. Sometimes it takes time for messages to settle in and your loved one may need time to reflect on what was said. And some people find that if they respond in the moment they might say something that is not intended or well thought out. Some people can formulate responses under emotional pressure, but most people can't. Remember, you have achieved your aim just by opening up the dialogue on a difficult subject.

Leah and Junaid have been in a relationship for six years and have gone for couples' counselling. One of the main problems was that Leah believed Junaid avoided having difficult conversations, but in reality, Junaid felt under pressure to respond immediately when Leah starting talking about "hot" topics (this is what we labelled the subject matter that was likely to end in arguments). It was established that Junaid would be happy to have these conversations but needed time to reflect and consider his thoughts once he had listed to Leah. They agreed to a have a "time out" once Leah had voiced her concerns so Junaid could reflect on what was said and to pick up the conversation the next day at a set time.

Do not expect to feel good after having difficult conversations. If the conversation has ended in a huge argument with you or your loved one storming out and slamming a door, then everybody will feel lousy. Sometimes you may feel relief for starting a conversation but frustrated by the end. Sometimes it could end well and you may feel hopeful and positive. You cannot predict how you will feel and it can be very up and down emotionally.

TIMING

Consider when you have these difficult conversations. In the morning when someone is rushing out the door for work or college, after a long day of study or looking after the children, or following a stressful doctor's appointment are not the best times to bring up your loved one's anxiety or obsessional problem. People are already feeling stressed and are possibly in fight or flight mode, so are unlikely to respond positively to what you say. You can time conversations to be more productive at different points in the day or week. So obviously in the case of anxiety and obsessional problems, if someone is very anxious and fraught with a looming trigger situation for them coming up, that's not the ideal time to have a conversation about changing a safety behaviour or treatment options. You can select a time when things are a bit calmer. Just don't avoid it! If there does not seem to be a "good" time, either create one or choose a time which is "less" tense. By choosing your timing to start difficult conversations, it doesn't mean that the situation won't escalate and result in an argument, but it will be less likely to happen.

SCHEDULING TIMES

It might be easier, especially in the case where someone is avoiding having difficult conversations, to "book" in a time to speak, so no one feels unprepared or confronted. You can also schedule times to carry on conversations if they are interrupted or become too heated, or if people want to have time to think about what is said. It ensures that people feel listened to, allows people to process what has been said and formulate a more even response. It also helps minimise the risk of the conversation escalating into an argument. It is important to acknowledge that you are thinking about things that have been said and that you're not just trying to avoid a difficult topic, it's just that that you don't have a response ready right now.

So, if you are having a difficult conversation with somebody, or it's a difficult topic for you, or it's too emotionally challenging, consider saying something along the lines of, *'I hear you. I need to think about this and process this. Can we speak about it again when I've had a bit of time to think about it? Perhaps in a day or two days.'* And suggest a specific time – *'How about 7.30pm tomorrow?'* Likewise, you can use this strategy and suggest another time to speak if your loved one needs to have some time to think about things too.

THINKING ERRORS

You or your loved one may have some thinking errors about difficult conversations which prevents you from being able to talk about their anxiety problem. For example, you might believe that having difficult conversations or arguments means that relationships are doomed (catastrophising), that people don't care or don't love you (mind reading), or that it's pointless having difficult conversations as nothing changes (crystal ball gazing). Refer back to thinking problems in Part One, Chapter Three and try to come up with more helpful ways to think about difficult conversations and their outcomes. Here are some examples:

UNHELPFUL BELIEFS ABOUT ARGUMENTS	MORE HELPFUL WAYS OF THINKING ABOUT ARGUMENTS IN RELATIONSHIPS
Arguments mean that the relationship is over.	Arguments are normal and do not mean the relationship is over. Everyone has them and we have not ended the relationship over previous arguments, so it is unlikely to end now. In fact, arguments allow us to air our differences and come back together stronger.
My partner doesn't love me because he disagrees with me.	It is normal and healthy to disagree with each other – it means you can learn from other people and review your ideas in life.
Nothing changes even if we argue about it.	Perhaps if nothing has changed yet, it means you should try another way of communicating and come at the problem another way. Eventually everything in life changes, whether you want it to or not.

THREATS

If you have a difficult conversation with somebody and they threaten to harm themselves or do something quite equally drastic, it can be very alarming. This is not your fault: you are not responsible for what they have chosen to say or do. It is a way of them showing their distress and possibly trying to stop the conversation or prevent implementing the changes you have outlined. Often it can be just a verbal threat because they dislike what is said or they are worried that because of the difficult conversation they are going to be abandoned or rejected. If you are concerned about them carrying out the threat, you act to keep everyone safe. You may need to ring emergency services and report it to the police and ensure that there are no dangerous objects around them.

Daly and Sue were trying to talk to their adult son Michael about his OCD problem. They wanted to explain that they didn't want to facilitate his OCD anymore but would be very happy to support his treatment for OCD. Every time they tried to have this conversation, their son became angry, accused them of not loving him and threatened to kill himself. Daly and Sue were extremely worried that he might follow through on this threat, particularly because he had a past of acting impulsively. On the advice of a psychologist they picked a time when Michael was less stressed and spoke to him calmly. When Michael made a threat, they said they would call the emergency services, and in fact did so when Michael kept repeating his threat.

Obviously in this scenario, Michael's parents would have preferred to not have had to call emergency services to the property. However, things do not always go to plan and they preferred to call emergency services and ensure their son was not going to harm himself, rather than take the risk – regardless of how small the risk was. Even if this damages the relationship at the time, you can work on rebuilding the relationship after you know your loved one is safe. And you do not want to be held hostage by this threat of self-harm.

By acting on their son's word, Sue and Daly were able to show Michael that they took him seriously and would not allow the threat of suicide to stop them from changing their behaviour. I must reassure you that in my experience these situations are rare, and even when they do happen, the relationships are repaired and people receive the urgent help they need in that moment.

Threats are not reasons to avoid difficult conversations. Because, again, if you are going to avoid conversations because you are concerned about the impact it will have on somebody, you will never have them.

USING PERSONAL PRONOUNS

During conversations it is best to use personal pronouns when describing how you feel and what you think. You are the one who feels the way you feel, behaves the way you behave, and thinks how you think. We are agents of our own actions and this is one of the basic philosophical tenets behind CBT. So, it is important to own your thoughts and feelings. For example, *'I feel/I believe/I think that...'* It's much less confronting to others and it is taking ownership over how you feel and think.

Imagine how you would feel if someone said the following to you: *'You always make this really difficult for the family. You never want to go out and you're ruining it for everybody.'* You would likely feel hurt, criticised and blamed. But if you heard the same sentiment expressed in a different way – *'I am really worried about you because we don't get to do things as a family. It upsets me that we can't seem to all go out and we miss having these special times together'* – you would be much more likely to think about what is said, reflect on the family time that you are missing, and more likely want to change it. In the second situation, the speaker is owning how they feel and what they think about it, rather than being accusatory. The speaker is trying to say the same thing in both scenarios – that they miss the family time together – but one way of expressing it is much more palatable and likely to receive a more positive response.

Here is another example of using "you" vs "I". The situation is a partner telling their loved one, who has panic disorder and social anxiety disorder, that they are frustrated by the impact on their life together.

Consider:

"You": *'You never want to go out and you always make things really difficult for me when I have to make up excuses to explain where you are. You always have a panic afterwards anyway and I hate what it's doing to us.'*

Versus:

"I": *'I worry when you get anxious and about the impact that's going to have on our friendship group. It makes me concerned that you are unable to see our friends and socialise and I don't like making excuses for you. I don't enjoy things the same way I used to with you and I think that's really sad because our relationship is really important to me.'*

Again, you can see that whilst the same message is being conveyed, the way it is phrased in the second one is more acceptable and therefore likely to be listened to.

Some helpful personal pronoun phrases are:
- 'I really care for you so...'
- 'I worry that...'
- 'I want the best for you.'
- 'I want to help you.'
- 'I feel frustrated when...'
- 'I hope things can be different.'
- 'I can see you're very distressed when...'
- 'I hear how you feel.'
- 'I understand your position. This is how I feel...'
- 'I don't blame you for...'
- 'I don't like it when...'

TAKING TURNS

It is also important to take turns speaking. I know this sounds very basic, but it is surprising how often I see people dominating the conversation and not allowing their loved one to respond or give their explanation or perception of things. Remember to pause and even ask your loved one if they have anything they want to say.

KEEP IT SIMPLE

Plan your conversation to cover a few points only – it may even help to note them down. Too much information will overload your loved one, particularly if they're feeling anxious. Try not to confuse the issue with multiple points – just pick out the few main ones you want to cover. We have all been in those arguments when someone says, 'and one more thing...'! Remember, it is not a good time to discuss your loved one's annoying eating or sleeping habits when you are trying to convince them to get help for their anxiety problems.

LOOK AT THE MEANING BEHIND WORDS

I always advise people to look behind the spoken words to find out what the meaning is and what the speaker intends. Remember that a significant amount of communication is non-verbal (some estimates are around 65%), so the words spoken are not the way we get our messages across. Most parents I know can silence their children with one look, and you know instantly from the way your loved one enters a room what mood they are in.

So, the spoken word is one way to get messages across, but not everyone is a sophisticated linguist. Some people are just better with words than others and can always seem to find the right words to say. Whilst you can be coached in this (think about all the politicians that speak but without saying anything meaningful at all!), you probably don't have the time, money or drive to do so. So instead, one tactic that can be useful is to look behind the words and see what is being communicated. It may surprise you. For example, a teenager telling their parents *'I hate you and wish you would leave me alone'* is normally really saying something along the lines of *'I am struggling in this hormonal and socially precarious world, and I am trying to develop my identity and independence. I would like some space to do this.'*

In the case of anxiety problems, words can disguise a loved one's anguish, fear or vulnerability. If your loved one picks a fight with you when they get home from a stressful, high-trigger day, it is often because it is the only space they have to let their feelings out and they are feeling scared and overwhelmed. If your loved one shuts down and doesn't say anything, it could be because they don't know how to explain how they feel and are confused by it all. I am not trying to let people get away with bad behaviour or poor communication, but it can help you to respond more effectively if you think about what is sitting behind the words, rather than the actual words or lack of words, as may be the case.

THE RELATIONSHIP UNDER THREAT

One thing that is often not verbally communicated is that people are fearful about the future of the relationship. This could be your or your loved one, or both of you. It is useful to reflect on whether this is true for you and, if this is the case, find a way to put it into words so that there is less ambiguity about how important the relationship is to you.

'I'm worried that this is going to impact on our relationship. It's really important to me that we have time together that we can both enjoy, and it's also really important to me that you are happier in life. I believe we can achieve these things if you get some good help and I want to support you in doing that.'

PUSH PAUSE

During a difficult conversation it is also okay to push "pause". But if you do that, do set a time or space for it to be picked up again – especially because you don't want people to think you're avoiding a difficult topic or that there will no follow-through on what is said. It's important for people to know they are being listened to and what they have to say is important to you. Try saying something along the following lines:

'I wanted to try to explain how my role is going to be different from what it has been, because I think I have not been helping you. I have been helping the anxiety problem instead. By how you've just responded it seems you're feeling very hurt by this, and I am sorry as I don't want to hurt you. I want the best for you, but maybe we should have a bit of time apart from this conversation, just to process things and let things settle, and then we can pick it back up again.'

PRACTICE HELPS

Like most skills in life, practising new communication skills will help you feel more confident using them and able to communicate more effectively. You can start by using some of these strategies in general conversation or when discussing minor problems – for example, if your loved one hasn't put the trash out despite promising to, or has not tidied up after cooking a meal. It is helpful to practise in low-emotive situations, and these skills can be useful in any communication, whether during a disagreement or not.

THERE IS NO PERFECT WAY

Despite your best efforts, there's no such thing as a perfect conversation. The goal is not to have a perfect conversation – the aim is to *have* the conversation and be able to talk about difficult things. It is okay if the conversation goes awry halfway through – we have all had the experience where we've tried to discuss an issue in a constructive and calm manner and then something has triggered us, resulting in someone saying something unhelpful and then having an argument. Remember the reason you are reading this book is because things are difficult already in your relationship and you are likely experiencing (or avoiding) conflict anyway. You are not going to make things worse, even with an imperfect resulting-in-an-argument attempt to communicate. If things become more difficult before they get better or there is conflict, at least something is changing. Change is better than things staying the same, and change is often accompanied by a period of discomfort or conflict.

CHAPTER SUMMARY

- Conflict in relationships is normal and difficult conversations should not be avoided.
- You can learn to be a more effective communicator and have difficult conversation by practising some communication skills:
  - Think about timing a difficult conversation for a less stressful time.
  - Take turns speaking to let everyone express their thoughts and feelings.

- Think about what your loved one is trying to communicate in their behaviour rather than just the words they use.
- Use personal pronouns to avoid making someone feel criticised.
- Practise communication skills on non-emotive topics.
- Pause the conversation and pick it up later if it becomes too emotional or argumentative.
- Keep the messages simple – aim to cover one or two points.

- If someone threatens to hurt themselves in some way, take it seriously and call emergency services if you need to.
- Difficult conversations don't end perfectly, but that is okay as the most important thing is to have them.
- Do not worry if the conversation is hard or ends badly as change often happens after periods of conflict.

CHAPTER THREE
STOP THE UNHELPFUL RESPONSES

As you now know, there are unhelpful things that you may have been doing without even realising it, such as facilitating avoidance, taking part in safety behaviours and giving reassurance that compounds the problem. Hopefully reading this book has helped you work out which ones you do. And now it is decision time – what are you going to do about it?

Be consistent

If you are planning to stop your unhelpful responses, then you must stop ALL of them, and remain CONSISTENT. This is very important! There is no point stopping "some" of the safety behaviours that you help with because the others then will become stronger and new ones could develop instead. It's like trying to collapse a structure – you need to take away all the supports at once for the structure to fall, otherwise it will become more dependent on the standing supports and precariously balance on them.

When you change patterns of behaviour, people don't like it because they are used to your old patterns and sometimes your new way of responding causes things to be more unpleasant for them. For example, if you used to give your toddler sweets at the checkout supermarket to keep them quiet, but then decided to stop that because you thought they were having too much sugar (plus it was expensive), then for the first few times you tell your toddler they are not getting sweets you will undoubtedly have a huge tantrum on your hands. If you remain consistent and do not give in, then in a few visits the tantrums will stop because your toddler will learn that no matter what they do, they will not be getting sweets. However, if you give in after two visits and give them sweets, then decide not to the following two weeks, then give in again… you will not only confuse your toddler, but you will have many more weeks of tantrums. These principles of behaviour change are the same for any behaviour – be consistent and stick at it. And be aware that you can get tantrums at any age – they might just look at bit different!

So, you will likely have some arguments, see increased distress and be accused of not loving your loved one or trying to make them worse. Like a toddler's tantrum, your loved one is just trying to figure out how to get their sweets (in this case, get their reassurance or help with their safety behaviour) but is usually able to hit out with their words rather than little fists and tears.

MAKE A PLAN

I recommend that you make a plan and work out what you are going to do to help your loved one and what you are *not* going to do (i.e. what you are going to stop doing). You can then share the list with your loved one and explain why you are changing these things. In order to help you with this exercise, I have provided a case study below as an example.

Sara's partner suffered from social anxiety disorder. After deciding she didn't want to facilitate his avoidance anymore, she told him that she would be going to social events they were invited to. And if he didn't feel like going, she would go alone. She also stopped giving him a lot of reassurance after a social event. Sara preferred to go out with her partner, but she also enjoyed going on her own and found that her mood improved too. Her partner used to be annoyed when she went without him, but she ignored his bad moods and over time he got used to it and the arguments stopped.

Below is Sara's action plan:

WHAT I (WE) WILL DO:	WHAT I (WE) WILL NOT DO:
Start going out to social events that I want to go to – alone if I have to.	Stop giving reassurance to the anxiety problem.
Invite friends and family over if I want to have them visit.	Stop making excuses for my loved one's behaviour or absences at social events.
Plan to go to the cinema once a month together and on my own if my loved one can't attend.	Stop avoiding social events because my loved one doesn't want to go.
Start exercising again – either together with my loved one or on my own.	Stop buying alcohol that my loved one uses as a safety behaviour.

Now, using the above as a guideline, you can write out your own action plan:

WHAT I (WE) WILL DO:	WHAT I (WE) WILL NOT DO:

When you discuss this plan with your loved one, you may not receive a positive response. That is fine, because you are not doing this to please them. You are doing this so you can give your loved one the best chance to acknowledge and recover from their problem. You are also changing your behaviour so that you can reclaim your life and stop letting someone else's anxiety or obsessional problem interfere in your life.

CASE STUDY
Kara's twenty-eight-year-old son had health anxiety. He was very worried that he might have a chronic degenerative illness and spent a lot of time seeking reassurance from her, visiting his doctor, and researching online. Kara found it exasperating and annoying and was worried she wasn't helping him by giving him reassurance and money for specialist appointments. After reading this (helpful) book, Kara decided to stop giving him money or reassurance – although she did offer to pay for therapy sessions for his problem. Her son was angry at her, but Kara felt relieved that she was doing the right thing and knew that over time their relationship would improve, especially if her son got the help he needed.

CHAPTER SUMMARY

- When you change your pattern of responding to someone, it is important to be CONSISTENT and stick to your plan.
- If you are planning on stopping facilitating safety behaviours, and avoidance, you must stop ALL of them.
- Make an action plan about what you are going to change and share this with your partner.
- Expect some arguments as your loved one will not necessarily like your action plan, but over time they will accept the changes and your relationship will improve.

CHAPTER FOUR
ASSIST YOUR LOVED ONE WITH BEHAVIOURAL EXPERIMENTS AND EXPOSURE TASKS

Let me tell you a story (trust me, the relevance will soon become clear):

Two lumberjacks employ a school-leaver to work with them in the forest. On his first day, they decide to play a prank on him by telling him to hold up a large, low-hanging branch of a tree which, they explain, is in danger of falling because it is so old. They say that they will come back with their tools to prune the smaller branches on the branch so that it does not fall off the tree. Then they walk off and leave him standing alone, supporting the branch. A walker comes along and asks the boy why he's propping up the branch.

'Because it will fall down otherwise,' he replies.

'How do you know?' the walker asks.

'Because that's what I've been told.'

Instead of laughing at him and carrying on, the walker suggests he takes one hand away from the branch. The boy is not keen because he's been told to hold it up and he doesn't want to lose his job on the first day. Neither does he want the branch to fall on his head. However, he takes the plunge and removes one hand, albeit tentatively. The branch doesn't move.

'Okay,' says the walker, 'why don't you take your other hand away now?'

'No way,' replies the boy. 'This might be the hand that stops the whole thing crashing down.'

'On the other hand,' replies the walker, 'that may not happen at all. It might just be that you're worried it will happen. Maybe you should try it and see?'

Gingerly, the boy removes the other hand. The tree remains as steady as it has done for the past 200 years. The boy looks at it. He is still anxious despite no longer holding the branch up.

'It's old,' he said. 'It could still just fall down. Or if the wind picks up, it could blow it down.'

'In that case,' says the walker, 'why don't you swing on the branch?'

The boy is very nervous. Of course he is – instead of supporting the branch, he is now going to do the opposite and try to make it fall down! He grabs the branch with both hands and begins to swing. Surprise, surprise – nothing happens!

Introducing behavioural experiments

This is a story I tell all my clients who need to do exposure (ERP) or behavioural experiments, as this analogy outlines the key reasons we need to do exposure or behavioural experiments when treating anxiety or obsessional problems. Behavioural experiments are ways of testing out whether unhelpful thinking is correct. In this story, the boy believed the branch was in danger of falling (his belief) and he was responsible for keeping it up and attached to the tree (his behaviour). The experiment was to test this belief out – and to do that he had to take a risk and let go of the branch. This is precisely what happens in anxiety and obsessional problems. People believe a feared outcome is extremely likely and therefore direct their efforts (their behaviour) to prevent this outcome from happening. BUT – and it is a big BUT – there is no evidence that the feared outcome will happen. It is in the future, and no matter what you say, you cannot predict the future.

Let's look at the vicious cycle of anxiety in this scenario:

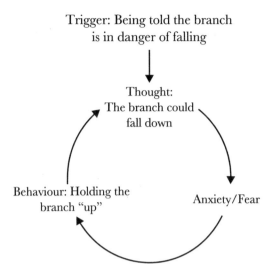

Trigger: Being told the branch
is in danger of falling

Thought:
The branch could
fall down

Anxiety/Fear

Behaviour: Holding the
branch "up"

By stopping his "safety behaviour" of holding the branch up –
and in fact trying to do the opposite by jumping on the branch
– the boy found out that his fears were indeed inaccurate and
very unlikely to be true. In the vicious cycle of anxiety, the
"behaviour" element was changed, thus providing the boy with
an exit route from the anxiety cycle.

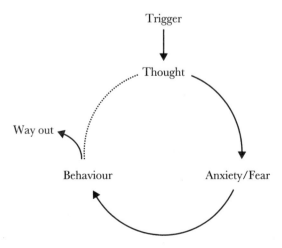

Trigger

Thought

Way out

Anxiety/Fear

Behaviour

In addition, the behavioural experiment also had the bonus of changing the boy's belief that the branch will indeed fall down and be his fault. This provides another route out of the vicious cycle of anxiety:

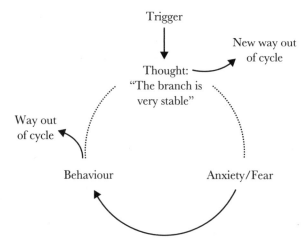

Exposure and Response Prevention (ERP)

The other form of behavioural experiment is Exposure and Response Prevention (ERP). This involves being exposed to the fearful situation and not being able to do a safety behaviour to alleviate the anxiety. An example would be in OCD if someone is worried about germs. An exposure exercise here could be to touch toilet door handles (the exposure) and then stop them from washing their hands (the prevention). The idea in ERP is that by exposing yourself to a threat, over time you will "habituate" to the anxiety until you get to the point where this trigger is no longer one of fear – it has become normal. Previously your loved one will have tried to avoid the fearful trigger or used a safety behaviour to make anxiety go away. But this does not change the fearful response; it only delays it until the next time the trigger appears.

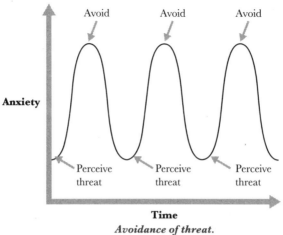

Avoidance of threat.

With avoidance we see that every time a threat is perceived, anxiety levels shoot up until it is avoided (or a safety behaviour is used) then it drops back down. Unfortunately, the next time the anxiety is triggered, it goes up again until the avoidance or safety behaviour brings it down – and so on, meaning that nothing is being done to reduce the fear and anxiety permanently.

This second graph shows what happens when someone is exposed to the fearful situation:

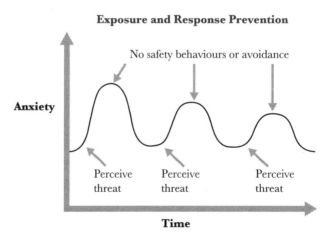

Exposure to threat and habituation of anxiety.

Now the anxiety decreases over time if you expose yourself to it. For example, say your loved one has a phobia around dogs, and their anxiety shoots up every time they see one. In normal circumstances they would run away to counteract the fear – but next time they see a dog the same thing happens again. However, if you are working with their dog phobia, you could bring a dog over to the house, and your loved one could stay in the same room as the dog. They are going to feel very uncomfortable, but I can guarantee that the next time you bring the dog in, they will still feel uncomfortable, but slightly less so. That's because they are now habituating to the threat (the dog), and each time you bring him in their anxiety will eventually lessen and will reduce much quicker over time. Your loved one's body and brain start to learn that the threat is not as bad as they thought, and that they survived.

'Okay,' your loved one may say, 'but I don't want to go near that dog in the first place, never mind be in the same room as it.' That's understandable; whatever the trigger is, their anxiety around it has been troubling them for a while, so it feels very strange and uncomfortable to suddenly stand up to it and see it for what it is. ERP contradicts everything your loved one has attempted so far to control their anxiety problem. They've avoided it or pushed it aside, using rituals and compulsions and safety behaviours, so it is a big ask for them to suddenly do the opposite and meet the threat head on. Hopefully they have had some help to challenge their unhelpful thinking and teach them about the anxiety process so they feel brave enough to start testing out whether their behavioural responses are keeping them safe. As you will see, they can start small and build up – such as being in the same room as the dog, but not having to touch it. The important thing is to ensure that the exposure situation is endured for long enough – say ten minutes or more. This is because people usually need ten to fifteen minutes for the anxiety fight or flight changes in the body to start calming down, so it is only then that they start to feel less anxious. Any shorter and leaving the room would be avoiding the situation.

Being a co-therapist

Undertaking experiments with your loved one is when being a co-therapist can be extremely useful. Not everyone will want someone to help them with experiments, but usually people do appreciate the support. When I am in clinic with clients, I always do the experiment with them. This is to both support them and further prove that there is very low risk attached to their fear, as it does not bother other people. This has led to some very strange and entertaining therapy sessions – from sitting on the ledge of London Bridge over the Thames, dangling our feet over the end (OCD), to yelling out 'I am a pervert!' at the top of my lungs (OCD), to vacuuming in a heated room whilst hyperventilating (panic disorder), to walking around the city with wet patches all over my trousers (social anxiety), to making "vomit"[xxii] and putting it around my office and the bathroom, to wearing my hair in pigtails and smeared lipstick while shopping (BDD and social anxiety) … The list is long, and seemingly weird to outsiders.

I am prepared to do something that makes me feel a bit uncomfortable to prove to my clients that there really is nothing to be afraid of – for example, running my hands over public toilet seats and then putting my hands on my face and hair. It would make anyone feel a bit squeamish, but rationally we know that the risk is very low and usually non-existent. I would just as likely catch an illness from the door handles at my local café. To me, thirty seconds of feeling uncomfortable for touching a public toilet seat – as opposed to three years of crippling OCD for my client – seems like a very small price to pay if I can help my client overcome their OCD. So it is okay not to love doing the experiments or to feel a little uncomfortable, but it is a small sacrifice to help your loved one overcome their problem.

Jordan *had checking OCD, in which he felt he had to check all appliances, outlets and the general security of the house multiple times. This took hours every evening and he often went to bed exhausted at 2 or 3am. He lived in* a small farming town, so there were no local psychologists and it took hours to drive into the closest city to see one. Jordan's sister lived in the same town and offered to work as a co-therapist for Jordan's treatment. The psychologist in the city advised them that experiments and exposures around the home would be best, and under the guidance of the psychologist remotely, Jordan's sister worked with her brother on his experiments. They were both delighted and relieved to see results in the first few tries, which motivated both of them to continue with the treatment plan.

PLANNING EXPERIMENTS

If you are planning to support your loved one by doing experiments with them, it is very important that you plan them properly. This is to make sure you are testing out their specific unhelpful belief. For example, if someone has a fear of dogs, taking them to a dog kennel may seem like a good idea, but if their fear is specifically of dogs unleashed and uncaged, it will not help challenge their belief that "unleashed dogs are very dangerous". Likewise in OCD, if someone is worried about causing offence to a deity (I have seen this form of OCD quite a lot), then taking them to a Christian church to purposely offend their god seems like a good experiment – unless, of course, they are Hindu and do not believe in a Christian god. So, it is important to ensure that the experiment is actually testing your loved one's belief and what they are afraid of.

DEVELOP A FEAR HIERARCHY

Sometimes it is very useful to develop a "fear hierarchy". A fear hierarchy is used in an exposure treatment plan and it lists out specific situations or feared stimuli that your loved one plans to face in their experiments. You start with an item that causes low-level anxiety and gradually work up the list until you reach the penultimate fearful situation at the top. Each item is given a rating (out of a hundred) of how distressing or anxiety-provoking the situation is.

Here are some examples below for Jen, who has BDD, and Kyle, who has social anxiety.

JEN'S LIST (BDD: WORRY ABOUT HER SKIN PIGMENTATION ON ARMS AND LEGS)	RATING	KYLE'S LIST (SOCIAL ANXIETY)	RATING
Wear a short, spaghetti-strapped summer stress.	100	Give a speech at brother's wedding.	100
Wear T-shirt and shorts to the park.	90	Plan a social event and attend.	85
Wear T-shirt and shorts together to cinema.	85	Talk to someone I don't know at bar or café.	85
Go out without using moisturiser or lightening creams.	80	Meet friends at a bar.	65
Wear shorts for a jog.	65	Go out to after-work drinks.	60
Wear T-shirt at cinema.	50	Invite a colleague to coffee.	50
Wear ¾-length trousers.	40	Tell a story at lunch.	35
Wear a ¾-length-sleeved top.	35	Eat lunch with colleagues.	25
Wear normal sunblock (not tinted sunblock) on arms and hands.	15	Speak at team meeting at work.	10

Some people find fear hierarchies useful and that they give them a structured way to work through their anxiety problem. Other people don't find them overly helpful and prefer to do experiments as the opportunity arises. I sit on the fence here – if my client likes them and it gives them the motivation to work through their anxiety problem, then I am all for it. However, I have also found that they give the idea that one situation will be significantly more anxiety provoking than others, whereas in reality, if people are doing behavioural experiments and exposure tasks, then they actually find the "higher" rating tasks are much less anxiety-producing than the first "smaller ones" once they reach them. This is because they have habituated to their triggers and they are starting to believe that the feared outcome is unlikely to happen anyway. Regardless, a hierarchy can be a very useful starting place and give people a sense of achievement as they work through the steps.

START SMALL

It is important to start small. You want your loved one to experience some success and feel proud of themselves to motivate them to continue. The first experiments and exposures are usually the hardest as it is the first time your loved one will have faced their fear head on, rather than avoiding it. Touching the door handle without washing their hands may seem small to you, but for someone with germ OCD it is a significant step forward. Not wearing make-up to go and buy a drink from the shop may be very easy for you, but it is incredibly difficult for someone with BDD.

PRAISE

Remember to tell your loved one how well they have done for trying a behavioural experiment and that you are proud of them. What they are doing is very difficult – facing their fear – and they are likely suffering from low self-esteem alongside the anxiety problem. This way, you give them some well-deserved credit and increase their motivation for trying new behavioural experiments next time.

Fiona had BDD and was worried about the shape of her ears. She would never leave the house without a hat and and spent hours styling her hair to cover her ears. One of her experiments was to push a very small amount of hair behind her ear when she went out to the shop and leave the rest of her hair covering her ear. This might seem a very small step to others, but it was a significant step forward for Fiona.

REPEAT THE EXPERIMENTS

A very important principle in behavioural experiments, especially ones that include ERP, is to REPEAT them. This is so people can habituate to the trigger situation, and then what they learn is reinforced. For example, someone with panic disorder who worries that they will panic on a train will feel incredibly anxious the first time they take a train trip, but by the fourth time they may only feel a little anxious, if they feel anxious at all. It is also better to repeat the experiment in a reasonably close time frame for habituation to occur. The person with panic disorder would be encouraged to repeat the experiment and take another train trip in the same week. If they didn't go on the train until three months later it would be unlikely that they would experience much, if any, reduction in their anxiety. It is also more likely that people will do it on their own when they repeat the experiment soon after completing it. In clinic I always set homework in which clients repeat the experiment between sessions on their own.

BUILD UP ON PREVIOUS EXPERIMENTS

It is easy to build upon previous success. If someone has a good outcome from a behavioural experiment, you can use the same experiment again but make it a little harder. People are more likely to be motivated to try an experiment if they had previous success in a similar one. For example, a person with panic disorder who did an experiment by taking a quick train trip from one stop to another, could follow up with the next experiment going between two stops and then three stops, and then they might be able to take a twenty-minute train journey.

LET GO

At some point you are going to have to step back and allow your loved one to do these experiments on their own because you could unknowingly become a safety behaviour (as in your presence reduces their anxiety), or your loved one may start to believe that they can't do the experiments without you being there and lack confidence in their own abilities. There is a delicate balance of support between helping in experiments and your presence becoming a safety behaviour. If you are unsure or suspect your presence is now a safety behaviour, you need to discuss this with your loved one. Eventually the goal is for them to be able to live an independent and successful life and be able to do all sorts of things on their own. If they resist doing things on their own, another option is to do *part* of the experiment with them. For example, if your loved one has a fear of catching public transport you could suggest, 'Why don't I do the first two stops on the bus with you and then get off, and you go one stop on your own? And I will meet you at that next stop when you get off.' Or they may choose to start a smaller step on their own, for example going one stop on the bus alone, even if they managed two stops with you last time.

Jacob had panic disorder and had been working through his fear hierarchy with his partner. When his partner suggested that they take a step back and let Jacob do some of the experiments on his own, Jacob felt very anxious and worried that he wouldn't be able to do it. His partner Aidan suggested that they set off together to the location of the experiment and he would then return home. Jacob could then come home after trying the experiment. Jacob still felt anxious but was confident that he could try the experiment and come straight back home to discuss the outcome with his partner.

WHEN THE BEHAVIOURAL EXPERIMENT DOESN'T GO TO PLAN

And this does happen. No one can predict the future, and no one can accurately predict the outcome of a behavioural experiment. That's the whole point of experiments – that we don't know what the outcome is going to be! Even if the experiment didn't go as planned, it is usually never as bad as your loved one imagined it could be and there is always something that can be learnt from the experiment. In my years of practice and experiments, I have yet to have one be such a disaster that it ended up making the anxiety or obsessional problem worse. In fact, even if the "feared" outcome did happen, it was never as bad as the client thought it would be. For example, a client with social anxiety had an experiment to talk to a stranger in a bar, and the stranger was very rude to him. My client was able to reason that the stranger was in fact not a very nice person, rather than it meaning anything about him personally.

Importantly, if things don't go as planned, you can still reinforce your loved one's efforts, rather than the outcome. I once took a client to go on a train ride to challenge his specific phobia of travelling on trains, but when we got to the station it was closed, and the trains were not running due to track problems. He was so anxious about it and had built himself up and was prepared to do it, so we were both very disappointed. But we used it as a learning experience about when things in life don't go as planned and that that is okay. We were able to take the train trip the following week.

In one experiment, a client had to do an activity without much planning and see what happened. She decided last minute to take her dog and her two children to the beach for the afternoon without planning it. Well, the dog ran away, the children lost their lunch boxes and it started to rain. Eventually the dog was returned by a fellow dog owner after it had tried to play with other dogs, and the children said they had an "amazing" time and thought it was very fun to play in the rain. Despite things not going to plan, the client believed the experiment was helpful as she now knew that she could cope better when unexpected things happened. She also felt proud that she had faced her fear.

HELPFUL DISTRACTION

Whilst your loved one is doing an experiment or is in the throes of an anxiety attack, it can be helpful to distract them from what is going on. This is not avoidance of the anxiety and triggers;

you are directly challenging the fear with the behavioural experiments. It is a way for your loved one to tolerate the anxiety rather than avoid it. The difference between avoidance and distraction is that avoidance is a problem in which people are effectively saying, *'I am not going to deal with this and will ignore it'*, whereas helpful distraction is when someone has already accepted they have an anxiety problem, is trying to deal with it and is CHOOSING to think about something else. For example, if your loved one has social anxiety and you are out with a group of friends at a social event, you may choose to discuss the unusual artwork or the architecture of the building with your loved one to draw their attention away from their anxiety. Likewise, if you are doing an ERP task with your loved one who has OCD, you may put on a TV show whilst they are resisting the urge to check something. They will still feel anxious, but it will help them let the anxiety subside – as we know it does in the habituation model.

A NOTE ON GAD

If your loved one has GAD then it could be hard to do the experiments with them, as a lot of their experiments and exposure will be to the worry process itself – for example, being able to sit with worrying thoughts and not respond to them, or resist giving in to the worry and seeking reassurance. Even if you cannot be part of the experiment, you can still encourage them to do experiments and be supportive. You might be able to offer practical help such as cooking dinner or doing the laundry or picking up shopping whilst they have some time to focus on their experiments. You can also take part in Applied Relaxation with them, which is a treatment strategy for GAD. Applied Relaxation is learning to relax quickly in trigger situations. I have discussed AR in more detail in the next chapter, as this is something you can do with your loved one.

Myron had GAD and was seeing a therapist about the problem. One of his homework experiments was to sit for ten minutes and allow the worrying thoughts to run through his head without trying to respond to them. Another homework task was to spend fifteen minutes each day doing progressive muscle relaxation exercises. Initially it was difficult trying to do these tasks as his three children kept interrupting him. After he spoke to his wife, Francisca, they planned things so that Myron could do this experiment in the evening whilst she either took the children to the park or played outside with them. This seemed to work well and Myron stopped worrying about whether he was able to do his therapy homework properly – one less thing to worry about!

REVIEWING AFTER THE EXPERIMENT

After completing an experiment, it is important to discuss with your loved one what happened, what can be learnt from it, and what can be done next time to build upon the completed experiment. Sometimes it can be difficult to reflect on it immediately afterwards as your loved one will still be very anxious after finishing it. But try to discuss it as soon as you can afterwards so the impact of the experiment is not lost. The things I ask my clients after they have done an experiment are:

- Did your prediction come true?
- How did you feel?
- If the outcome was not as you predicted, what does this mean for you now?

- What do you conclude from this experiment?
- What is your anxiety problem trying to tell you now?
- How can you challenge this with another experiment?

Here are some examples of feedback from people who did experiments set for homework:

In the case of dog phobia, an experiment of walking in the park around dogs.

Did your prediction that dogs would run up and jump all over you come true?
No.

How did you feel?
Very anxious that I would be attacked by a dog and relieved it didn't happen.

If the outcome was not as you predicted, what does this mean for you now?
I should stop worrying!

What do you conclude from this experiment?
That I need to stop the worry as it is very unlikely that a dog is going to attack me.

What is your anxiety problem trying to tell you now?
That even if it is worry, how do I know that I won't be attacked by a dog in the future when I go to a different park?

How can you challenge this with an experiment?
Visit different parks and walk around them, especially in the morning or evening when people are likely to be walking their dogs.

In the case of social anxiety, an experiment of giving a presentation at work.

Did your prediction come true that you would make a mistake and be too embarrassed to continue?
No.

How did you feel?
Very anxious and worried that I would make a mistake during the presentation and that people would notice and think I am not fit to do my job.

If the outcome was not as you predicted, what does this mean for you now?
I should stop worrying!

What do you conclude from this experiment?
That I can do presentations despite feeling anxious, and that I won't necessarily make a mistake.

What is your anxiety problem trying to tell you now?
I might make a mistake next time I do a presentation.

How can you challenge this with an experiment?
Volunteer to do more presentations, and even make a small mistake on purpose and see what happens.

CHAPTER SUMMARY

- Behavioural experiments are an essential part of treatment for anxiety and obsessional problems.
- Behavioural experiments are meant to challenge unhelpful beliefs, so it is important to stop safety behaviours to test out whether a feared outcome is going to happen.
- Exposure and Response Prevention (ERP) is a type of behavioural experiment for anxiety and obsessional problems in which someone does not perform a ritual or compulsion in response to a trigger.
- Habituation is when anxiety reduces over time when you are frequently exposed to the feared trigger.
- Taking on a role as co-therapist can be very helpful for your loved one and you can take part in the behavioural experiments to support them.
- Repetition of experiments is key to building up confidence and ensure habituation occurs.
- A fear hierarchy is when you approach the lesser anxiety-provoking situations first and then work up to the most fearful situation.
- In GAD it might be difficult to take part in the behavioural experiments because they can often focus around a person's worry process, but you can offer practical support in other ways so they can focus on their therapy homework and experiments.
- Review the experiment after it is completed so your loved one can reflect on what happened and build on their success.
- Experiments don't always go to plan, but they always offer a learning experience and are rarely (if ever) as bad as your loved one predicted.

CHAPTER FIVE
HELP YOUR LOVED ONE WITH APPLIED RELAXATION

Applied Relaxation (AR) is a treatment technique developed in the 1970s as a treatment for phobias and panic disorder[xxiii] and later as a treatment for GAD. Whilst over the years CBT has replaced AR as the recommended treatment for phobias and panic disorder, AR remains an effective treatment for GAD. AR involves identifying situations in which anxiety is likely, noticing the early warning signs of feeling extremely anxious, and then learning to relax the body quickly – as in twenty to thirty seconds. As part of the physiological response to anxiety the body becomes tense, and a feature of GAD is muscle tension, muscle aches and pains. When you are feeling anxious and stressed you may notice feeling tense or clenching your teeth until your jaw feels tight. You may experience upper or lower back pain or that your shoulders become tense.

One of the main techniques in AR is Progressive Muscle Relaxion (PMR), which involves tensing and relaxing muscle groups systematically and overcoming some of the physical symptoms of anxiety. The good news is that anyone can do PMR and it can be a really useful way to relax your body, even if you aren't feeling all that stressed. So you can give it a go with your loved one, encourage them to do the exercise, or even do it without them if you find it helpful! You could read the script for them or set aside some time for them to go and practise whilst you cook dinner. It is only a short exercise; it won't take long and your loved one can still help with the washing up!

It is not a standalone treatment for other anxiety problems as they still need the cognitive restructuring and behavioural experiments, but it can still be used to help people relax when they are feeling stressed. In all other disorders apart from GAD, AR could become a "safety behaviour" and prevent people from facing their fears, so I would not suggest using it in lieu of cognitive restructuring, behavioural experiment and exposure tasks.

MUSCLE TENSION SCAN

If you are not sure whether you hold your muscles tense when you are stressed or anxious, it can be useful to "scan" your body next time you are feeling stressed to see what areas feel tense or tight. Think about where you often feel tension and "tightness" in your body – you may have noticed that certain parts of your body feel tense now whilst reading this book, especially if you have had a stressful day.

PARTS OF THE BODY TO CHECK FOR TENSION

- Forehead
- Shoulders
- Lower legs
- Mouth and/or jaw
- Arms
- Neck
- Back
- Chest
- Legs

Do not worry if you can't feel tension in your body right now though; this is just to help you to start thinking about it. So next time you are feeling stressed or anxious, scan your body and see what you notice.

PROGRESSIVE MUSCLE RELAXATION (PMR) SCRIPT

I have provided a script below that I use for PMR. In sessions I ask my clients to record this exercise on their phones as we do it, then practise it at home every day. It only takes five minutes to do, and once you can do it without the recording, you can reduce it to the main muscle groups and it will only take thirty seconds. So, I suggest you record this onto your phone or device which plays through a speaker first before doing the exercise.

I also ask my clients to stay sitting on their chair whilst they do the exercise. People naturally think they should lie down; however, in real world situations how many times are you lying down when you feel very anxious or stressed? It is much more likely you will be sitting or standing, so it is better to practise in these physical positions you will be in when you are most likely to feel stressed. When you are first practising it is also helpful to remove any big distractions such as TV or music, although again in the real world you will likely be in nosier environments when you feel stressed. I would also suggest not doing this exercise immediately before going to sleep – the goal is not to induce sleepiness but to learn to systematically relax your body to reduce anxiety tension.

GENERAL PROCEDURE FOR PMR
- Start by slowing down your breathing.
- When you start, tense each muscle group for five seconds.
- When you are tensing the muscles, make sure you can feel the tension but not so much that you feel a lot of pain.
- Relax the muscle group for ten seconds.
- When you have finished the procedure, remain seated for a few moments, allowing yourself to become more alert.

RELAXATION SEQUENCE ADVICE

I have written the script below so you can record it for yourself or your loved one. When talking, use a soft voice and slow pace. For the five deep breaths, allow enough time for someone to slowly breathe in before counting up to five. After tensing each muscle group, pause for five seconds. Then after relaxing each muscle group, pause for ten seconds.

Below is the script (the writing in the brackets are instructions for you. Do not say these out loud):

- Take five deep breaths.
- Breathe in... breathe out... (say this five times).
- Focus on your right hand and forearm. Make a fist with your right hand... (pause for five seconds)... now relax... (pause for ten seconds).
- Now focus on tensing your right upper arm. Bring your right forearm up to your shoulder to "make a muscle"... (pause for five seconds)... now relax... (pause for ten seconds).
- Focus on your left hand and forearm. Make a fist with your left hand... (pause for five seconds)... now relax... (pause for ten seconds).
- Now focus on tensing your left upper arm. Bring your left forearm up to your shoulder to "make a muscle"... (pause for five seconds)... now relax... (pause ten seconds).
- Now to your forehead. Raise your eyebrows as high as they will go, as though you are surprised by something. Hold it... (pause for five seconds)... now relax... (pause for ten seconds).
- Now squeeze your eyes tight shut... (pause for five seconds)... now relax... (pause for ten seconds).
- Open your mouth as wide as you can, as you might when you're yawning... (pause for five seconds)... now relax... (pause for ten seconds).
- Now focus on your neck. Put your neck forward and then pull your head back slowly, as though you are looking

up to the ceiling... (pause for five seconds)... now relax... (pause for ten seconds).

- Tense the muscles in your shoulders as you bring your shoulders up towards your ears... pause for five seconds)... now relax... (pause for ten seconds).

- Focus on your back and shoulder blades. Now push your shoulder blades back, trying to almost touch them together, so that your chest is pushed forward... (pause for five seconds)... now relax... (pause for ten seconds).

- Breathe in deeply, filling up your lungs with air. Hold it... (pause for five seconds)... now relax... (pause for ten seconds)

- Squeeze your buttock muscles and hold them... (pause for five seconds)... now relax... (pause for ten seconds).

- Now to your thighs and legs. Tighten your right thigh... (pause for five seconds)... now relax... (pause for ten seconds).

- Now onto your right lower leg. Pull your toes towards you to stretch the calf muscle and hold... (pause for five seconds)... now relax... (pause for ten seconds).

- Now to your right foot. Curl your toes downwards. Hold... (pause for five seconds)... now relax... (pause for ten seconds).

- Tighten your left thigh... (pause for five seconds)... now relax... (pause for ten seconds).

- Now your left lower leg. Pull your toes towards you to stretch the calf muscle and hold... (pause for five seconds)... now relax... (pause for ten seconds).

- Now to your left foot. Curl your toes downwards. Hold... (pause for five seconds)... now relax... (pause for ten seconds).

- Now relax your whole body... (pause for ten seconds).

- And take five deep breaths whilst you focus back on your surroundings...'

- (Finish)

If you have tried this, I am sure that you found it relaxed your body. Now the most important thing to do is practise. This is so the skill becomes ingrained and you or your loved one can use it whenever you need to. Once you or your loved one has practised the full PMR technique, it can be cut down so you can practise tensing and relaxing the parts of your body that need it.

CALMING YOUR BREATH

This is one of my favourite exercises. It is the simplest technique to try to calm yourself down. By calming your breath, you are taking a moment and telling your body to calm down. It is a great thing to use when you feel yourself getting upset, angry, stressed, or frustrated.

Imagine you walk into the bathroom after a long and very busy day to see that somehow creatively your child has managed to block the drain in the shower (just to see what happens) and has flooded the whole bathroom in an inch or so of water. Cue a calming, deep breath! Combining the calming breath technique with a quick muscle relaxing exercise is a shorter method to relax your body in times of stress and tension.

Use your nose to breathe in and your mouth to breathe out.

- Start by noticing how your breath feels as you inhale and exhale slowly.
- Now try to slowly make each inhalation longer by drawing your breath down towards the abdominal area in a smooth and steady fashion.
- Pause briefly and notice again the slow and steady way in which your breath is released as you exhale.
- Now that you are paying attention to your breath, you can start the counting rhythm.
- Breathing in slowly, count 1... 2... 3... 4... 5.
- Now hold for 1... 2...

- Breathe out for 1... 2... 3... 4... 5.
- Try to maintain this slow, even, controlled rhythm in your breathing by continuing to count in your head for at least 10 breaths.

CHAPTER SUMMARY

- Muscle tension is a common symptom of GAD and anxiety.
- Applied Relaxation is a way to relax your body during moments of anxiety or when you are anticipating stress.
- Progressive Muscle Relaxation is a specific method of reducing muscle tension in which you systematically tense muscle groups then relax them.
- Other methods of AR include breathing exercises, and shorter versions of PMR.
- Anyone, including you, can benefit from practising these exercises and it is especially helpful for people diagnosed with GAD.

Please note that breathing can be very useful when people are feeling anxious, but it should not be used instead of CBT.

CHAPTER SIX
TAKE A BREAK FROM THE ANXIETY PROBLEM

Anxiety and obsessional problems can be overwhelming and can dominate life. I have worked with people and their families when it seemed that their whole lives operated around the anxiety or obsessional problem. On the other hand, people can have anxiety and obsessional problems that only rear their head occasionally, and outside these moments life can continue as "normal". I remember one gentleman who came to see me for help with relationship problems and it became clear that he actually had OCD, although it was mild and unrelated to the problem for which he came to therapy (for interest's sake, we tacked on a handful of sessions at the end of this therapy to target the OCD problem, which was resolved successfully).

REMEMBER WHO YOUR LOVED ONE REALLY IS

It can also seem that your loved one and the anxiety problem are merged – that one does not exist without the other. But this is not true. Your loved one is a person with their own personality, beliefs, values and opinions. They have their own interests, hobbies and unique ways of expressing themselves. It may seem like the anxiety problem has taken over your loved one, but underneath they are still there. The funny, charismatic, sensitive, basketball-playing, amateur-painter Comicon fan is still there amongst all the other stuff. It is really helpful to remind yourself of this and try to spend time with your loved one outside of the anxiety problem.

I used to see partners and families in clinic and it seemed like their relationships all revolved around the anxiety and obsessional problem. The people suffering from the anxiety problem felt lost and believed their whole identity was defined by the anxiety or OCD or whatever problem they had. When they were making headway in treatment, I had to help them define who they were once the anxiety or obsessional problem had resolved, and to rebuild their relationships with their partners and families.

Your loved one did not choose to have this problem and it is not their fault. You may feel annoyed or frustrated with them a lot of the time, especially if you think they are not trying to get better. No one actively chooses to suffer from crippling anxiety or an obsessional disorder that makes going outside impossible. Try to remind yourself of who your loved one is without the anxiety or obsessional problem. Who was it who you enjoyed spending time with? If it is your partner, who was it who you fell in love with? If it is your child, who was it who you dropped off for their first day at school?

Make a list of all the things that you like or love about your loved one. You can even include the qualities that are a bit annoying and endearing, things that they like doing or hate to do and things that you did together, so you have a full picture of your loved one. I have provided a case study below as an example and to help you think of your own.

Susie's husband Matthew has OCD. Whilst lately it seems like it is taking over their relationship, Susie wanted to remind herself of who the man was that she fell in love with, so she made the list below.

Matthew is to me:
- *A loving partner*
- *Generous to me and others*
- *Proper in his behaviour and always polite*

- *Someone who likes to eat Chinese food whilst drinking beer*
- *A man who loves horror movies (which he knows I hate!)*
- *A person who hates being late for things and when people don't fill the kettle up after they have used it*
- *A fitness fanatic who loves getting up early for exercise*
- *Someone who laughs at my silly jokes and thinks my dancing is hilarious (I think it is pretty good)*
- *Someone with whom I like to take walks and hiking holidays*
- *Someone who agrees with me that Christmas is too commercial and prefers to keep it simple*

Now try your own list.

After doing this activity you will hopefully feel more positive towards your loved one. It can be emotional reminding yourself of their qualities and the things they enjoyed or did when they were younger. You may feel nostalgic for the past or sad that you don't see this side of your loved one very often anymore. You may feel surprised about the things you had forgotten you liked or admired about them. But you will feel differently towards your loved one after this exercise, rather than just frustrated, irritated or annoyed.

I am hopeful your loved one can recover from their problem and be all these things without the anxiety or obsessional illness, but until this point, there are still other things you can try to have a more positive relationship with your loved one.

TAKE TIME OUT FROM THE ANXIETY PROBLEM

Talk to your loved one and agree to have a "time out" from the anxiety or obsessional problem once a week. This is where you can forget about the impact of the anxiety or obsessional problem for a short time, or even pretend it is not there. This is not avoiding the problem or saying it doesn't matter, because as we know avoidance is not helpful and the problem *is* significant. But you can still have enjoyable time together with your loved one DESPITE the anxiety problem.

This means not discussing the problem, treatment or therapy, and no exposure experiments (though it would be great if they naturally occurred). You could take a trip out somewhere, play computer games, bake or do some gardening – whatever it is that you both enjoyed doing once.

Giovanni's best friend Jay *has panic disorder with agoraphobia. Giovani is frustrated that Jay won't come out with him to hang out like they used to and he knows that Jay's parents are pressuring him about getting help for his problem. Giovanni has arranged with Jay to go to his apartment once a week for a movie night. They stream a new movie and eat nachos and chat about things without talking about the anxiety problem. They both really enjoy it and Jay always feels more positive and motivated to get treatment after spending this time with Giovanni.*

MAKE A POSITIVE MEMORIES BOOK AND PUT UP PHOTOS

This is another way that you can remind yourself of the times you and your loved one used to enjoy before or despite their anxiety problem. You can go through photos or other reminders of your relationship such as artwork or crafts (in the case of children), ticket stubs, or special occasion cards. You can also write stories or memories. If you are into collages or scrapbooking, this could be an activity for you. But if not, you can download a lot of applications that make it exceptionally easy to make a photo book or memory book.

Stephanie's husband Fred *has GAD and in the last few years he has become more and more anxious and worried. Stephanie has found it hard to remind herself of what made the relationship special in the first place, so she decided to make a positive memories book. She put in photos from their wedding and holidays, old Valentine's Day cards she had saved, ticket stubs from concerts they enjoyed and other special mementoes from their relationship. Once she had finished, she shared it with her husband*

Fred. He was so touched by seeing it and reminded of the value of their relationship that he agreed that he would get some help for his anxiety problem.

Likewise, finding and putting up photos of you and your loved one around your house or apartment can have a similar effect. It is a small thing to do, but having constant reminders around you of times when you were happy or when things were not so difficult can have a positive effect on your mood and remind you that things can be different.

You also never know what the impact of these exercises could be. it may help your loved one's mood if they suffer from depression, and these types of activities are a first step in the treatment of depression. It could help motivate your loved one to get help or try harder in their therapy once they remember how great the relationship can be when unfettered by anxiety or obsessional problems. It can help show your loved one how much you care, despite having to make the other changes we've discussed in the book such as cutting out safety behaviours and/or stop taking part in rituals or compulsions. There are many unintended positive consequences that could happen once you invest a bit more in the person and stop giving the anxiety and obsessional problem attention.

CHAPTER SUMMARY

- The anxiety or obsessional problem can make it hard to remember the uniqueness and special qualities of your loved one.
- The qualities, values, interests and irritants that make up your loved one are still there – you just have to find ways to remind yourself (and them) of this fact.

- You can make a list to remind you of who your loved one is outside the anxiety problem, put up photos of a happier time, and/or create a positive memory book.
- You can also have an official "time out" from the anxiety problem and enjoy spending time with your loved one.
- Positive consequences of doing these things could be to motivate your loved one to get help and improve their mood.

CHAPTER SEVEN
LOOK AFTER YOURSELF: MAKING SURE YOU ARE CAPABLE OF PROVIDING SUPPORT

In the safety briefings on airplanes you are told that you must put on your own lifejacket and breathing apparatus before putting them on those dependent on you. Obviously, this is because in order to ensure the safety of those more vulnerable, you need to be breathing and alive to do it. The same principle applies when you are looking after people with mental health problems – you need to be capable of providing the assistance they need. This means you need to be as resilient, physically well, emotionally stable and mentally strong as you can be. Providing support or care for someone with an anxiety or obsessional problem can be demanding, and for those people caring for someone with a severe problem which renders them housebound, it is even more taxing. So, to be supportive, compassionate, empathic, and potentially working as a co-therapist, it is important for you to remain positive and look after yourself.

> It is not selfish to prioritise your own wellbeing. It is imperative.

Think about it this way: if there are two people in a relationship who are struggling with their mental health, both people are neglecting their physical health and both are socially isolated, the relationship will deteriorate and neither person will receive the support they need. In contrast, take one person who is suffering from poor mental health who is being supported by somebody else who is able to maintain their own wellbeing. This scenario is more likely to result in a positive outcome for both people, as the unwell individual will be helped to achieve better mental health.

Often people do not look after themselves as well as they could due to exhaustion. They feel guilty investing in themselves when their loved one is suffering from an anxiety problem. But the guilt is misplaced. You are not doing this because you are selfish or don't care for your loved one – you are doing this because you do care and you want things to be different. For things to change, you need to be in a healthier space to allow them to be different. It is also not selfish to enjoy parts of life, to do activities that give you enjoyment or a sense of achievement, even if your partner or family member is unable to. In fact, it is vital for mental wellbeing and can be preventative against developing a depressive illness!

It is very important to invest in your own wellbeing in order to be able to promote wellbeing to others. As psychologists we constantly peddle the message to clients that health and mental health are interlinked and equally important.

In this chapter I cover the basic features of looking after yourself – those that we all know we should do. I also discuss other avenues of support specifically for people caring for those with anxiety and obsessional problems that can provide an outlet as well as practical advice.

EXERCISE

I cannot even begin to list the research studies showing the positive results of exercise on your physical and mental health. Exercise is beneficial for so many reasons and shown to improve wellbeing and general health, including weight management, cardiovascular health, improvements in mood and self-esteem, memory, concentration and much more.

So, the take-home message here is DO SOME EXERCISE.

It is recommended that adults take about thirty minutes of moderate exercise a day – it could be walking quickly to work or to the supermarket, running around while playing at the park with your children, playing a team sport, walking up the stairs to your apartment or at work, cycling to work or school, walking with friends, and so on. It does not have to be training for a marathon or competing at the Olympics. You can easily build it in to your day. If anyone says, 'I don't have time for exercise' I would strongly disagree in most cases – the minimum recommended amount of exercise is three and a half hours out of a whopping 168 hours a week – roughly 2% of your time (or around 3% of your waking hours in a week, generously accounting for eight hours of sleep a night!). I spend a reasonable chunk of my "exercise" time running around with my children at playgrounds or chasing them whilst they zoom around on their scooters. You can build exercise in to suit your life – just make sure you do.

EATING WELL

Like exercise, there is a wealth of information on healthy eating and the importance of a balanced diet for longevity of life, physical wellbeing and good mental health. There is some fascinating research linking good mental health with the types of food you eat and how they interact in your gut with bacteria and microbes.[xxiv] It would be hard to list all the research findings and recommendations, so I have attempted to summarise briefly:

- Eat lots of fruit and vegetables
- Eat unprocessed foods
- Cut down on sugar and salt (they hide in a lot of processed foods!)
- Eat lots of fibrous food including legumes and wholemeal grains
- Moderation is key with alcohol and caffeine
- Eat a variety of foods
- If you eat meat, eat lean meats a couple of times a week

I don't subscribe to diets or restrictive food eating, such as cutting out all chocolate, because the evidence suggests that diets do not work as people eventually put on the weight they lost (plus more) once they stop the diet (And anyway, dark chocolate in small amounts can have a positive impact on your digestive system). Also, cutting out entire food groups often leads to an unhelpful cycle of bingeing and restricting. Balance, variety and moderation are key. If you have problems eating well you need to think about why, because the solution will be different for each problem.

For example:

- If you struggle with a healthy diet, have a one-off appointment with a nutritionist to get more information around good meals.
- If you overeat emotionally (including binge eating and eating because of boredom) see a psychologist for help with managing your emotions.
- If you "don't have time" invest in a slow cooker or spend a week practising healthy and quick meals. (I have become a bit of an expert in this of late whilst working, writing this book and looking after my young children!)
- If you think you cannot afford to eat healthily, be creative and research. There are a lot of excellent money-saving blogs by people focusing on food and eating well without spending a fortune.
- If you have digestion problems, see a doctor and change your diet around – for example, trial being a vegetarian or vegan for a week.
- If you can't "cook" (most people – those that are mobile or have the ability to be active in the kitchen – can cook; it just takes some practice!) enrol in a cooking course and borrow some easy recipe books from the library.

These are just a few of the reasons people give for not eating well. But all these reasons – and the others – can be resolved with some creative problem solving and the motivation to change.

SLEEP

Sleep is an important factor in maintaining wellbeing. There has been a wealth of evidence recently that we need good quality sleep to be healthy and it turns out most of us are not getting enough. Many of us are in jobs that require long hours and responding to emails outside of "official" work hours. Most of us are continuously connected to a form of media and lots of people are addicted to their phones and social media. It all takes a severe toll on our sleep. So, one basic step of wellbeing is to ensure you are getting enough sleep, and the right quality sleep at that.

I have seen many clients who are have very disrupted sleep cycles due to their anxiety or obsessional problem. In OCD, it is common for people with checking or cleaning rituals to be up all night completing their rituals and people with co-morbid depression will often have disrupted sleeping patterns. People with anxiety can suffer from insomnia and can have trouble sleeping due to uncontrollable worry. In fact, sleep problems are one of the diagnostic criteria in GAD.

So you may have a partner or family member whose nocturnal patterns or tossing and turning are keeping you awake. Maybe you lie awake, restless and worrying about your loved one. You could be not sleeping well for many reasons (late night online shopping or checking out Facebook are just two). Whether you are not getting enough sleep or not getting good enough quality sleep, what I am going to tell you is not going to be new or revolutionary. You probably know it already, but you need to have better routines around sleep.

WHAT IS GOOD QUALITY SLEEP?

There are various definitions of what "good quality" sleep is, but a generally accepted definition is:

- Sleeping most of the time while in bed (at least 85% of the total time you are in bed)
- Falling asleep in thirty minutes or less
- Waking up no more than once per night

- Being awake for twenty minutes or less after initially falling asleep[xxv]

If you are reading this and have small children, then you are probably not getting good quality sleep, although this will hopefully pass as the children grow up. Also, night waking for adults is very normal and everyone does it as part of a standard sleep cycle. The problem of night wakenings is when you fully wake up and cannot get back to sleep quickly. To make it more likely that you will have good sleep, basic sleep hygiene like the tips below can help.

TIPS FOR BETTER SLEEPING

- Have a sleep schedule with the same bedtime and wake-up time every day. This helps to regulate your body's internal clock.
- Try a relaxing bedtime routine including a warm shower, as this increases your body temperature and helps you prepare for sleep.
- Avoid napping in the day.
- Exercise daily.
- Try to ensure your sleep environment is not too hot or cold and that it is free from noise and light.
- Use bright light in the morning and during the day to help manage your circadian rhythms. Avoid bright light in the evening.
- Avoid alcohol, cigarettes, and heavy meals in the evening.
- Wind down. Your body needs time to shift into sleep mode, so avoid electronics and spend the last hour before bed doing a calming activity such as reading.
- If after going to bed you still can't sleep, go into another room and do something relaxing until you feel tired.

It may be the case you have to change your sleeping arrangements in order to get some sleep. For example, if somebody is up being very anxious or obsessional very late at night, you don't have to be up as well. Try telling them,

'I know that you're distressed and it's very difficult for you right now, but I need to get some rest so I can go to work tomorrow and get the children up and ready for school.'

If you continue to have trouble sleeping, please see your doctor to discuss medication options. You might consider trying an online CBT sleep programme.

SOCIALISING AND CONNECTION

Human beings thrive on social connection and prosocial interactions. Many studies have shown the link between reported levels of happiness and positive social relationships.[xxvi] We like to feel like we belong and to interact with other people, but sadly these days loneliness has become a problem for many people. Loneliness is associated with a myriad of health problems. There are different theories on why loneliness is on the rise, including the loss of community, capitalism, the rise of the internet and advancement of robotics. Loneliness is likely the result of a complex interaction of many factors.

Why is this relevant for you? Well, in my experience, families and partners of clients with anxiety and obsessional problems can feel cut off and isolated from friends and families and struggle to find the time to socialise due to the extra demands of caring for someone with an anxiety problem. You may have stopped socialising because you feel guilty or because you don't want to go without your loved one and leave them at home alone. You may worry about their wellbeing when you are gone. Or you may even be too tired to bother trying to socialise. Whatever the reason, it is important that you now build social connection back into your life. Your loved one may be upset or resentful or have FOMO,* but they will be okay.

You can try inviting them to come along with you – *'I'm meeting up with Jose and Fred tonight. We are going to see a comedy show together because we haven't caught up in a long time. Would you like to come?'*

Or, if you are going out alone, you can say something like, *'I'm going away for the weekend to this swimming event. I haven't done that for a*

---

* FOMO is the phenomenon known as the "fear of missing out".

long time, and I know it's going to be difficult being on your own, but I'll call once a day to check in with you.'

Unsure of how to start this process? Volunteer at a local charity. It will offer you the chance to meet others, do something positive for your community and offer meaningful social connection. If you are not quite ready for that step or live in a rural area but would like to connect with others, you can join online forums and write a blog. The internet offers an excellent way to connect with likeminded people if you are unable to get out and meet face to face.

MINDFULNESS

You will probably have heard about mindfulness, and you may even know what it is or have learnt some techniques yourself. Mindfulness is about being in the present moment, not caught up with the past or worrying about the future. Have you ever noticed that when you are doing familiar and repetitive tasks, like driving or washing dishes, your mind is often miles away, thinking about something else? You may be thinking about a work call or worrying about some upcoming event. Whatever you are thinking about, you are not focusing on your current experience, so you are not properly in the "here and now". So, mindfulness is the opposite of this – to be aware of present-moment sensations, thoughts, and feelings without judging them and just allowing them to be. Sounds idyllic? Well, it is actually good to be mindful amongst our current increasingly switched-on and frantic world.

Mindfulness is an extremely useful tool to reduce negative thinking and distress and you may find it helpful to build it into your life. It is a skill that can take time to develop, and like any skill it requires effort, time, patience, and ongoing practice. Mindfulness can be taught in a number of ways and attending a mindfulness group has been shown to be one of the most effective methods for learning it. You can also find many online resources and apps for mindful exercises – try a few before settling on the ones you like, as there are lot to choose from.

The core features of mindfulness are:

Observing
Directly experiencing things through your senses rather than being analytical. A natural tendency of the mind is to try to think about something rather than directly experience it. Mindfulness teaches you to move your attention away from thinking to simply observing thoughts, feelings, and bodily sensations.

Describing
Noticing the details of what you are observing. For example, if you are observing something like a raisin, the aim is to describe what it looks like – its shape, colour, and texture. You can also apply this description process to non-tangible things like feelings; for example, emotions can be described as "heavy", "tense", "strong" and so on.

Participating fully
Taking in the whole of your experience and trying to notice all aspects of the task or activity you are doing, with your full care and attention.

Being non-judgemental
Being accepting of your experience and not trying to avoid or control your experience. Not judging means not classifying experiences as good or bad, right or wrong. This can be one of the more challenging aspects of mindfulness and can take some practice.

Focusing on one thing at a time
When observing your own experience, focus your attention on one thing at a time, from moment to moment. It is normal for

distracting thoughts to emerge while observing but try not to follow these thoughts with more thinking. If you have drifted away from the observing and sensing mode into thinking mode it is not a mistake. Just acknowledge it has happened and then return to observing your experience.

IS MINDFULNESS HELPFUL FOR ANXIETY PROBLEMS?

I included mindfulness in this chapter for you, the person who is supporting their loved one, not as a treatment for your loved one's anxiety problem. I am always asked by my clients whether mindfulness is useful in the treatment for anxiety disorders. The confusing answer is "yes and no".

Yes, because mindfulness helps us to have experiences without judging them – so if you are caught up in a rumination cycle, it may help break the uncontrollable worry by allowing you to sit back and observe the worrying thoughts without attaching any meaning to them, thus avoiding the associated anxiety.[xxvii] So it can be useful for people who have GAD and worriers who do not meet the criteria for GAD.

No, because mindfulness may prevent people from challenging the cognitive processes (the unhelpful interpretations) that are part of the vicious cycle of anxiety. And even more problematic is the fact that mindfulness may become a "safety behaviour" itself and prevent people from facing their fear. If when they need to be exposed to the anxiety-provoking trigger they instead try to distance themselves from the experience by being "non-judgmental" and "observant", this effectively becomes avoidance of the anxiety. A good example of this is someone with panic disorder (like those in the below case study) who finds it difficult to go on trains and buses. If they use mindfulness apps on their phone to "zone out" and distance themselves from the experience, they may feel less anxious, but they're also not facing their fear and instead they are taking part in a safety behaviour. If they can't access that app for any reason one day, their anxiety will be worse, because, as we know, avoidance is unhelpful and keeps the problem going!

Theo has panic disorder and finds it very difficult to go on trains and buses, which – as he does not have a car – are his only means of transport. He read about mindfulness and has been attending a local mindfulness group. He has been using the sayings as "mantras" and when he has to take the bus to work, he "zones out" and plays mindfulness exercises from an app to mentally distance himself from his experience. It works as he feels less anxious, however, this means that Theo is not actually facing his fear and is just cleverly avoiding facing the anxiety. The mindfulness has become a safety behaviour. When he forgets his headphones or his phone runs out of battery, he feels even more anxious than he used to.

So, my general advice is that perhaps for GAD and those who are worriers, mindfulness could be useful. If your loved one has a phobia, panic disorder, social anxiety, OCD or BDD, then I would suggest that they have proper CBT treatment first. Then they can add mindfulness as a tool for general wellbeing after completing treatment – very much like yoga, sport, eating well and sleeping betterr. But *you* can do mindfulness! It is a very valuable skill to help with stress, and if your loved one has an anxiety problem you will undoubtedly feel stressed at times. So please try it and build it into your life if you find it works for you.

DEPRESSION AND ANXIETY

A lovely couple came to see me in my clinic. The husband had moderate OCD which started worsening due to a trigger event on a holiday six months previously. During the assessment it was clear he needed help quickly to stop his condition deteriorating further. However, it also became obvious that his wife was struggling too. She had found the situation very stressful and had become depressed. Had she not joined her husband for part of the appointment (if I can, I usually ask family members for their input as they provide helpful perspective) I would not have known she was depressed, nor would she as she had put down her exhaustion and low mood to caring for her husband. I advised her to get some help and address her depression, which I believe she did. Her husband improved significantly in treatment with me, and when treatment was finishing, his wife accompanied him for the final appointment. She was brighter in mood and more positive, and both were excited about the future.

So, if you are feeling down or anxious and it is causing you problems, it could be that you have depression or an anxiety problem of your own. It may have occurred in the context of caring for someone with an anxiety problem, or their anxiety problem may be a contributing factor combined with other reasons. It doesn't really matter at this point why you are depressed or anxious; what is important is that you seek help for yourself. It can be easy to dismiss symptoms as tiredness or stress, but if you haven't felt yourself for at least a few weeks, please see your doctor as you may need your own treatment and therapy. As a bonus, your loved one will see you getting help and it may encourage them to do the same.

MAKE A SELF-CARE PLAN

Now take a moment and think about your own wellbeing. Make a list of the areas in your life that need help and why you think they are problematic for you. Now consider what you could do to improve these areas. They may be easily solved, or perhaps you need some time to think about the best way forward. As long as you have identified the areas that need help and reasons why they are problematic, you have taken the first step towards changing them.

I have included a case study below to give you guidance.

Jayne's daughter, Fay, has social anxiety disorder. Fay has just started working part time after finishing school but is finding it a struggle. Jayne accompanied her daughter to a psychologist appointment to see how she could help her. During the appointment the psychologist asked Jayne several questions about her own wellbeing, and it became obvious that Jayne suffered from generalised anxiety disorder (GAD). Her daughter Fay said she wasn't surprised as her mother was such a worrier. Jayne actually felt relieved as she had been worrying more than usual lately about Fay and was not sleeping well. Jayne started seeing her own therapist and was trialling a medication to help. Jayne was still able to support Fay in her treatment but felt better supported herself.

Jayne's self-care plan:

MY PROBLEM	WHY THIS IS A PROBLEM	WHAT I AM GOING TO DO ABOUT IT
I worry about my daughter all the time.	Turns out I have an anxiety problem myself!	CBT therapy.
I experience poor sleep.	I can't get to sleep as I am worrying too much.	Hopefully learn some strategies in CBT to help with sleep and stopping worrying.
I feel tired and physically exhausted all the time.	I'm not getting enough sleep.	Try some exercise and hopefully the CBT will help.
I'm not seeing friends.	I feel too tired/can't be bothered.	Contact Carla and see if she wants to meet for coffee.

Now have a go at writing and problem solving your own self-care list. You can be creative and put down multiple solutions. Just make sure the solutions are realistic and achievable – there is no point putting down that you will run an hour a day if you currently don't exercise at all. You are more likely to accomplish a goal for fast walking for fifteen minutes. Accessing your own therapy may be too expensive at the moment if you are paying for your loved one's treatment, but joining a mindfulness group or group support sessions could be more affordable (besides, there is good evidence that mindfulness is best delivered in a group format).

MY PROBLEM	WHY THIS IS A PROBLEM	WHAT I AM GOING TO DO ABOUT IT

SUPPORT GROUPS

You may want to connect with other people going through a similar experience and there are support groups set up for friends, family members and partners of those suffering from mental health problems. They offer a chance for you to meet up and share your experiences and provide practical support and tips. Online forums can also be helpful and charities often provide support forums or a network of people who are in a similar position. Charities also provide several valuable services including advocacy, annual conferences for members, helplines and information courses for family members.

CHAPTER SUMMARY

- Your wellbeing is important and you need to prioritise your own mental and physical health so you have the resources to look after your loved one.
- The basics of positive wellbeing are eating well, exercising, good quality sleep, socialising and connecting with other people, and looking after your mental health.
- Mindfulness teaches people to be aware of their surroundings, focus on the present, and not to judge or get caught up in unhelpful thinking patterns. It is a good tool to use for general wellbeing, but it is recommended that if your loved one has an anxiety disorder other than GAD, they receive CBT treatment before using mindfulness.
- It can be easy to make excuses for not looking after yourself, but you can reflect on what areas of your wellbeing are suffering and make a plan to improve these by setting achievable and realistic goals.
- If your own mental health is deteriorating, you may need therapy and medication. You can be a role model for your loved one by acknowledging you need help and accessing treatment.
- Charities, support groups and online forums can all provide advice and support for those caring for someone with an anxiety or obsessional problem.

CHAPTER EIGHT
DEPRESSION AND BUILDING ACTIVITIES BACK IN

I have written this chapter from the perspective of your loved one having depression, but the advice is applicable for you too if you are suffering from depression. It is normal to experience clinical depression as a result of problematic anxiety and depression can equally affect those caring for their loved ones with mental health problems. So, if you have been feeling more down than usual, or think you might be depressed, the information in this chapter may be useful for you as well as for your loved one.

Depression is the second most common mental health problem after anxiety disorders,[xxviii] and many people experience depression in their life for all sorts of reasons. So, if after reading this chapter you think you may be depressed, do not feel ashamed – remember it is a very common illness and there are very good treatments available to help you feel better.

WHAT IS DEPRESSION?

Depression is defined by having low mood for more than two weeks, plus **five** of the following symptoms:[xxix]

- Feeling tearful and hopeless
- Reduced interest in pleasurable activities
- Significant weight gain or loss
- Insomnia or hypersomnia (sleeping too much or too little)

- Sluggishness
- Feeling tired
- Loss of energy
- Feeling worthless or excessively guilty
- Not being able to think
- Inability to concentrate or make decisions
- Thoughts of suicide

While we may all experience some of these symptoms from time to time, if you or your loved one has had low mood consistently for the past two weeks and at least five of the other symptoms, then you or they are probably depressed. Some people find the "thoughts of suicide" symptom worrying and frightening, but it is a reality that in depression people can often experience these types of thoughts. I would be very concerned if your loved one wanted to kill themselves and found comfort in these thoughts, or has made a plan to kill themselves, or had tried to kill themselves in the past. If that were the case, I would ask you to seek professional help for your loved one immediately.

However (and slightly confusingly), I am not talking about intrusive thoughts about suicide as part of OCD. I have worked with a number of people who have had intrusive thoughts about committing suicide and therefore worry that they want to kill themselves and are at risk of doing so. The difference in this situation is that the intrusive thoughts cause intense anxiety and lead to the person avoiding any situations in which they worry they may cause themselves harm. In contrast, in depression, thoughts of suicide do not lead to this extensive avoidance or reassurance seeking, and the thoughts don't cause as much anxiety and fear as found in OCD.

There are other types of depression that people can get alongside an anxiety problem, including persistent depressive disorder (PDD)[xxx] (previously known as dysthymic disorder), which is a persistent but slightly less severe low mood. If you have persistent depressive disorder, your mood will have been low for most of the day, more days than not, for at least two years. Alongside the low mood, you will have two of the following symptoms:

- Low appetite
- Low energy
- Low self-esteem
- Poor concentration
- Feelings of hopelessness
- Difficulty making decisions

This depressive illness may not have the same symptom severity as major depressive disorder, but it is chronic and can be helped with treatment. Depressive disorders are debilitating and can affect the recovery process from anxiety and obsessional problems. So, if your loved one is also depressed alongside their anxiety problem, it could be expecting too much of them to be fully engaged in treatment for their anxiety. Think about it – if you're feeling down and hopeless, you are not sleeping well or eating properly and your motivation is barely existent, you are unlikely to be ready for the challenge of treatment designed to meet your fears head on! But the good news is that if your loved one tries the treatment strategies for depression, it is likely that their depression will lift enough for them to start treatment for their anxiety problem.

MEDICATION

Your loved one may benefit from medication to help lift their mood. A lot of medication used to treat anxiety is also prescribed for depression, so there may be an added benefit to taking an antidepressant. However, if your loved one is taking medication, they will still need to have psychological treatment for their anxiety problem. Medication is a useful starting point for those people who are anxious and depressed, and research suggests that it can be a useful way of kick-starting recovery. Some people are reluctant to take medication for depression or anxiety, but even though depression is a mental health problem rather than a physical one, medication can be an important stepping stone in the right direction. If someone had chronic diabetes or a physical injury, they wouldn't question that medication has its place. That said, not everyone with depression needs medication, and there are other strategies to help that can help lift someone's mood.

BUILD ACTIVITIES BACK IN

When someone has depression, they often have stopped doing the things they used to enjoy. If they used to swim regularly, go to a dance class or a pub quiz, or meet up with friends after work, they may now find excuses to go home and sit in front of the TV. Depression depletes energy, enjoyment and the sense of achievement you get from things, and in turn this starts a "vicious cycle" – very similar to the vicious cycle of anxiety – of not putting any effort into doing things, therefore getting nothing out of the activity. To help change this vicious cycle, your loved one can use what I call a "Behaviour Booster".xxxi This is essentially doing activities to get some enjoyment or a sense of efficacy or achievement.

Let's look at a case study to put this into perspective.

Janet has an anxiety problem and recently she has also been feeling really down. She used to go swimming a few times a week before work and found this really helped reduce her overall anxiety, but she has started to miss these swimming sessions as she feels too tired, can't be bothered and doesn't seem to enjoy them anymore. Janet has become depressed alongside having an anxiety problem.

Using a scale, we can see what has happened to Janet.

Before Janet was depressed, she enjoyed swimming. She found it easy to make time for it and get to the pool and felt proud of herself afterwards.

BEFORE DEPRESSION

Janet scored 8/10 on the enjoyment scale and 7/10 on the achievement scale, whereas it took little effort (3/10) to motivate herself to go swimming.

Before I felt depressed, I enjoyed swimming (8/10).

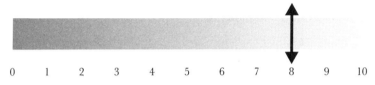

Before I felt depressed, it took me little effort to go swimming (3/10).

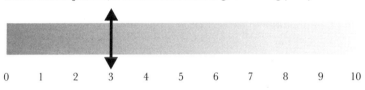

Before I felt depressed, I got a sense of achievement after going swimming. (7/10)

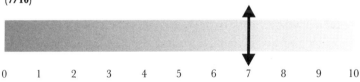

Now let's look at the same scale during the onset of Janet's depression:

DURING A DEPRESSED EPISODE

When I am depressed, I get less enjoyment out of swimming (3/10).

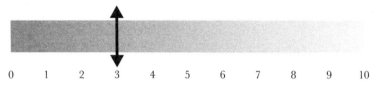

When I am depressed it takes much more effort to go swimming (8/10).

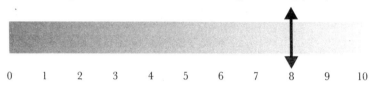

When I am depressed, I get only a small sense of achievement after going swimming (5/10).

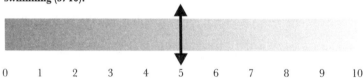

Now you will see that some of the scales are exactly the opposite – that Janet got little enjoyment from swimming, felt she had achieved less (perhaps she swam only half the distance she normally would), and she had to make a much bigger effort to actually get to the pool. This is what happens when people are depressed – they stop doing the things they enjoy as it takes so much more effort to get such little enjoyment. Their activities feel less effective and it hardly seems worth it to them, so they stop doing the activity at all.

So, if we examine the situation now, in the middle of Janet's depression when she can't be bothered to go swimming, let's see what happens:

When I am depressed, I avoid doing things I enjoyed. I get no enjoyment out of life. (0/0).

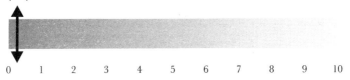

| 0 | 1 | 2 | 3 | 4 | 5 | 6 | 7 | 8 | 9 | 10 |

It takes no effort to avoid things (0/0).

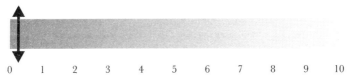

| 0 | 1 | 2 | 3 | 4 | 5 | 6 | 7 | 8 | 9 | 10 |

I get no sense of achievement from doing nothing (0/0).

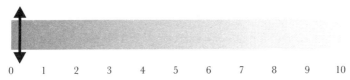

| 0 | 1 | 2 | 3 | 4 | 5 | 6 | 7 | 8 | 9 | 10 |

Janet is not getting any enjoyment or a sense of achievement from swimming at all, so she continues to avoid it. But look again at the middle graphs at the onset of depression where she is getting even a little enjoyment and sense of achievement from swimming, despite being depressed. This is what often trips people up – they think that as they only experience a small amount of enjoyment or get less of a sense of achievement from an activity compared to what they used to, why bother doing it? BUT a small bit of enjoyment or feeling like you have achieved something is better than having no enjoyment at all and feeling ineffectual. In addition, the research tells us that doing this activity is often enough to lift someone out of a depressed mood on its own.[xxxii] So a "Behaviour Booster" is about planning a few activities ahead – nothing too heavy or too taxing, but small things that help people reconnect with the pleasures they once enjoyed and to feel effective again. If your loved one is suffering from depression, this is precisely what they need to be doing.

You may have already noticed that if you are trying to get your loved one more active or encourage them to do some activities, that they seem brighter and uplifted at the end of it. You will know yourself that some days when you feel like you can't be bothered doing things – whether it is a sport, exercise, or socialising – that if you force yourself to do it anyway, you rarely ever regret it.

BE A CO-THERAPIST

This is another area in which you can be a co-therapist – by encouraging your loved one to do a "Behaviour Booster", or even doing it with them. You can help plan one with your loved one and discuss it with them afterwards to see how beneficial the "Behaviour Booster" was. I ask my clients with depression to fill in the following sheet to help plan their "Behaviour Boosters". I ask them to select activities that they used to enjoy, or ones that gave them a sense of being effective or achieving something:

DESIGNING A BEHAVIOUR BOOSTER

My activities this week are:

I plan to do these activities on the following days at the following time (e.g. Wednesday afternoon):

What help do I need to do these activities (e.g. a friend's company, childcare, getting a lift)?

After the activity, describe how it went below. How much effort did it take? How much enjoyment did you get from it? Did you get a sense of achievement?

Mark your rating from 1 to 10

Enjoyment [　] Effort [　] Achievement [　]

For example, Janet's answers could look like this:

My activities this week are:
Swimming twice a week for twenty-five minutes.

I plan to do these activities on the following days at the following time:
Monday and Thursday before work.

What help do I need to do these activities (e.g. company, childcare, getting a lift)?
It could help if my partner went to the gym at the same time then I would have some company on the way.

After the activity, describe how it went below. How much effort did it take? How much enjoyment did you get from it? Did you get a sense of achievement?
It went well – I didn't swim as far as I used to, but I managed thirty lengths, which is more than I thought. I felt tired but really pleased that I had done it and it made me feel better all morning.

Mark your rating from 1 to 10

Enjoyment [3] Effort [8] Achievement [4]

Just like with the exposure experiments for anxiety problems, it is beneficial to review the "Behaviour Booster" soon after completing it. If your loved one enjoyed the activity and felt better after doing it, you want to ensure that they record and remember feeling like this before they start to feel depressed again. And please remember, whilst I have written this exercise for your loved one, it is equally applicable to you if you too are suffering from low mood.

TACKLING THINKING PROBLEMS

Another strategy in helping lift a depressed mood is to analyse any thinking problems. I have already referred to these as they relate to anxiety problems (see Part One, Chapter Three), but they can apply to depression too. For example, Janet might have been "catastrophising" or "jumping to conclusions": *Oh, I can't be bothered going to the pool today; it's absolutely pointless as I won't enjoy it.* You can see that if that's how she was thinking, she was unlikely to attempt to go swimming at all. A better way of reviewing this way of thinking is to subject it to some simple but effective questioning:

1   Is it **100% true** that there is no point going to the swimming pool whatsoever?
    No, as I haven't even done it yet so I don't know what the outcome will be.

2   Is it **helpful** to think about it this way?
    No, because it's stopping me doing things.

If the answer is "no" to either of these questions, it opens up the possibility of looking at the situation another way. Perhaps Janet will say to herself instead, *'Okay, I have some days when it all feels overwhelming, but I did enjoy swimming a bit last time and I felt better afterwards, so I may try again this week.'* Every situation can be viewed multiple ways and quite possibly there is no "right" way. For example, two people walk past you in the street and burst out laughing. You may think, *maybe they're laughing at me?* or *that guy sounds like he told a hilarious joke* or *he must be intoxicated as there is nothing funny going on around here*, and so on. There are many ways you can interpret the event, and the way you interpret it will depend on how you are feeling, previous experiences and mental frameworks called schemas.* You can choose to go with your original explanation that they are laughing at you, which would cause you to feel self-conscious and anxious. But you can also choose to see it a different way too, a way that could be a truer representation of the reality of the situation. So now there are two more questions you can ask yourself.

> **Are there any thinking problems in my thoughts?**
>
> **Is there another way of viewing this situation?**

The new way of thinking about the event doesn't have to be perfect because life is not perfect and things can often be difficult. But even so, there are still many ways to think about events. For example, Janet may acknowledge that she is feeling down and things are difficult at the moment, but that there is hope that things will be different if she tries an activity: *I know I am feeling low and it is really hard work getting to the pool, but there is a chance I will enjoy it even a little, which is probably worth the huge effort to go!*

If it is your loved one who is suffering from depression, they will hopefully get more help with challenging these thinking problems with their psychologist or therapist, but it is helpful to know about

---

* A schema is a cognitive framework or concept that helps organise and interpret information. Schemas can be useful because they allow us to take shortcuts in interpreting the vast amount of information that is available in our environment.

thinking problems in depression as you may be able to gently challenge some of their unhelpful interpretations. It can be very easy to get stuck into patterns of thinking that are pessimistic and not be able to see a way out of the negative cycle. Sometimes if other people give you a different view it can change your viewpoint, or at least reinforce the idea that there are multiple ways to see events and that your view is not always the correct one or, indeed, most helpful.

CHAPTER SUMMARY

- Depression is a very common mental health problem and many people with anxiety and obsessional problems also have depression. Those caring for someone with a mental health problem can also suffer depression.
- It can be very problematic if it prevents your loved one from being able to engage in treatment for their anxiety or obsessional problem.
- Depression can lead to suicidal thoughts and plans to commit suicide. If you believe your loved one is at risk of harming themselves or trying to commit suicide, you need to seek help urgently.
- There are good treatments available for depression including CBT therapy and medication. Medication may also help alleviate the symptoms of your loved one's anxiety problem.
- The first step in treatment for depression is to do a "Behaviour Booster". You can work as a co-therapist by encouraging your loved one and making plans to do an activity together.

- People experience thinking problems in depression so it is helpful to challenge these and to try to see things from another more helpful perspective
- If you or another family member who is caring for your loved one are depressed, the strategies and advice in this chapter will help you too. Please also see your doctor to discuss treatment options.

PART THREE
MOVING ON

GETTING ON WITH LIFE DESPITE THE ANXIETY PROBLEM

So, at this point you may be seeing your loved one working through their anxiety problem, or you could still be despairing that they are not acknowledging it is a problem and refusing some or all forms of help.

Whatever your loved one is doing (or not) with regards to their anxiety problem, life will continue. It is not going to wait until they decide to get help and receive treatment. It will not wait until they have completed treatment. Life is going on as you read this book – and you need to be proactive in the life you want to lead. Until now, you may have believed that you weren't able to make future plans until your loved one's anxiety problem resolved, felt guilty thinking about your future, or worried that your future plans may not co-align with your loved one's future plans. But it is time for that to change – you need to get on with your life DESPITE your loved one's anxiety problem.

In practice, this means no longer putting off things that you want or need to do to get the future you want. In earlier chapters I asked you to think about what activities you were no longer doing due to your loved one's anxiety problem. Now I am asking you what goals or plans you have side-lined, put on hold or changed because of your loved one's anxiety or obsessional problem. It could be moving house, taking a holiday, studying, losing weight, or going for a promotion. It could be something that you have thought about for years or a relatively new opportunity, such as a promotion at work or travel.

Peter wants to retrain as a physiotherapist. He is currently a personal trainer and he wants to go back to school and study towards a degree. His girlfriend has health anxiety and is currently going through a "bad" period. She has never had treatment, but once the "bad" period is over, she says she is better and doesn't need help… until the cycle repeats itself. Peter has put off studying as he was worried that he wouldn't cope with the stress and time demands of study if his girlfriend was going through a "bad" period because he would still need to work in his current job alongside studying. However, he has spoken with his friends and family and decided that he would like to start the course now, so he has enrolled at the local college. He has explained to his girlfriend that he is going to retrain and that he may be less available during that time due to him being very busy and often studying late at the library.

I understand why you may have put things on hold – we would all prefer the timing to be "right" to make changes or embark on new adventures, especially if there is an element of risk involved or if the changes affect others – for example starting a family, moving countries, or quitting your job to start your own business. All changes or big plans involve an element of uncertainty – the outcome is unknown. We naturally try to minimise the possibility of a negative outcome by making plans and ensuring the rest of our lives are as organised as they can be.

However, this is a fallacy. There is no such thing as the "right time" and periods of big change can often occur due to external reasons (and often stressful ones). For example, many more people are self-employed and running their own business now, (which is more unpredictable financially), because people were "forced" into working for themselves due to redundancies in the financial downturn of the global economy. That is not to say that people do not want to be working for themselves – it may be the best decision they ever made in their working lives – but it was preceded by a period of stress and uncertainty. Likewise, many people wait for things to line up in life before having children, such as finding a suitable like-minded mate, getting married, making

good progress in their careers, financial stability, buying a house…
However, life rarely ever works like this. If you are waiting for all
these things to happen first, you could miss the opportunity to
have children.

Similarly, if you are waiting for your partner or loved one to
change and get better from their anxiety problem, you might
be waiting a while. There is often no clear or definite end to an
anxiety problem, unlike finishing a course, training for a race or
event, or saving X amount of money, all of which have a defined
finish point. Waiting for your loved one to get better is just another
example of waiting for the "right time", which does not exist. So,
in summary, don't wait. Start making those plans now.

WHAT IF MY LOVED ONE GETS VERY DISTRESSED OR ANGRY?

This could happen. What you are doing is not selfish – it is self-
determining. You are setting out to achieve your own goals and
desires in life and taking control of your own destiny. I am not
suggesting you do this to the absolute detriment of everyone else
and everything – and unless you were a sociopath, this would
be very hard for you to do! But I want you to think about your
own future and what you want to achieve and to start putting the
wheels in motion towards these plans. It could be that you want to
go travelling next year, or on a camping trip next month. It may
be starting a new course or hobby, or training for a marathon.
Whatever it is, you can start now. Your loved one wants you to be
happy and fulfilled, even if their anxiety and obsessional problem
is getting in the way of them saying this. Once you have explained
to your loved one that this is your plan, they may get upset and
feel that you are excluding them. You can reassure them you are
not, and in many cases, you would prefer them to be part of your
plans. For example, if you want to take a family holiday, you want
your loved one to be part of it too. If they become angry or upset
when you talk about your future, it could highlight to them what
they need to change in order to be part of your future plans.

You are not doing this to hurt your loved one. You are doing it because you have your own goals and desires in life and you deserve to have the opportunity to realise these.

WHAT IF MY LOVED ONE GETS WORSE OR IT AFFECTS OUR RELATIONSHIP?

Let us be clear about one thing – if your loved one's mental health deteriorates in the face of change, it is not you making them worse. Your desire to achieve your goals and have new experiences is not going to make your loved one's health deteriorate.

What may make the anxiety and obsessional problems worse is the inaccessibility of safety behaviours or reassurance. For example, if you went travelling around Europe for six weeks and left your adult son, who has moderate to severe OCD, at home, you might remove the ability for them to seek reassurance from you or engage in some rituals or other safety behaviours. He cannot call you to "check" something or seek your reassurance that everything will be okay. He possibly will feel more anxious and may seem worse on your return. But this only proves that you were in some way propping up his anxiety problem, and the full extent of it is only now being seen.

I cannot promise that it won't negatively affect your relationship. But if that is the case, it would also negatively affect your relationship if you didn't try to achieve your own goals and desires in life. You would start to feel resentful and angry, and relationships do not thrive if one partner is feeling this way. It may be your relationship was in trouble before the anxiety became problematic and you feel guilty for leaving your partner whilst they are mentally unwell. If it is a family member, please remember conflict is normal in family dynamics, and I would be surprised if the conflict was new and not a repetition of unhelpful communication patterns. It is also much harder for a family member to estrange themselves, and if they do, it will be the result of a multitude of factors, not just you making plans for your future. Whatever the case, your relationship may suffer, but it likely will have suffered anyway regardless of you taking this step. Relationships are complex whether or not someone has an anxiety or obsessional problem, so if your relationship ends, it will not be just because your partner suffers from an anxiety problem.

Gerald was in a long-term relationship with Naomi. He really wanted to get married and start a family. The only problem was that Naomi suffered from emetophobia (fear of vomiting) and GAD. She was reluctant to get treatment as she was very fearful that any medication options would make her feel nauseous, which was precisely what she was trying to avoid! As well as being very worried about the exposure exercises she had read about in CBT treatment, the problem was that she would not consider getting pregnant due to the morning sickness associated with pregnancy. Despite being together for four years, Gerald gave Naomi an ultimatum – either get help for her emetophobia or he would end the relationship. Sadly, the relationship ended, but Gerald did find a new partner in a few years and was able to start the family he wanted. Naomi eventually got treatment for emetophobia as she realised it was preventing her from achieving the things she wanted in her life.

WEIGHING UP PROS AND CONS

If you are still undecided about whether you should follow your own dreams and future plans, it might be helpful to consider the pros and cons of doing so. This is a commonly used CBT technique that can help people decide which path to follow. As the name suggests, you list all the pros of behaving in a particular way and then all the cons, before stepping back and reviewing the list. Sometimes the act of writing these down and seeing the list makes it very clear for people what they should be doing. Below is a case study that provides an example.

David is nineteen and lives at home. He has OCD and panic disorder and finds it exceptionally difficult to travel on any form of transport. His parents want to take a family holiday at Christmas with him and his two siblings, but they have been worried about whether David can come with them. They have not had a family holiday for four years and would like to give the children some new experiences. After explaining this to David, they book flights for their trip – including a seat for David. However, on the day David decides he cannot travel and stays at home. His parents are disappointed but know that David is capable of looking after himself. David is angry at his family for "leaving" him at Christmas, but he also knows that he is really angry at himself. He thinks of what his future will look like if he doesn't get help and get better.

David's parents' pros and cons list for going on holiday:

PROS	CONS
We would really like a holiday – it has been four years since our last one so it would be nice to have a break.	David may not be able to go and will feel left out.
Our younger children deserve to have a holiday and it would be good for them to have fun.	If David does not join us, we will worry about him a lot.
If David can come it would be good for him to be in a new environment.	The other children will miss David and he will not be part of the family holiday.
If David cannot come, it will give us all a break from the OCD.	
We will only be going for a week, and can return quickly in the case of an emergency.	

As you will see, in this list the cons column is predominantly about their loved one's anxiety problem. If you take out all the cons related to your loved one's anxiety problem, it would be interesting to see what items you have left on this list. It could be sobering to think about the plans you have on hold due to your loved one's anxiety problem. Alternatively, you may see that it is an only minor feature in the decision-making process and other factors weigh more. Whatever the outcome, a pros and cons list can be a rational aid to help you think about why you have put some life goals or future plans on hold.

If you have your own personal decision to make, write the pros and cons in the table below:

PROS	CONS

COMMUNICATION

As always, it is important in relationships to communicate clearly and effectively. If you are planning to make some changes in your life and take steps towards these goals or plans, then I encourage you to speak to your loved one. You may find it helpful to review the communications chapter before speaking with them about your plans. Be clear about what your plans are, what you want to achieve, and that you are doing this for yourself.

CHAPTER SUMMARY

- You are an individual with goals, desires and future plans. It can be easy to put these on hold when your loved one suffers from an anxiety or obsessional problem.
- There is no such thing as the "right time" to make changes and put plans into action.
- There is no clear or defined end if you are waiting for your loved one to get better from an anxiety problem.
- Your plans to work towards goals or make future plans may cause your loved one some distress and affect your relationship, but relationships are complex regardless of the anxiety or obsessional problems, and it will cause problems in your relationship if you *don't* work towards your own goals.
- It can help to write a pros and cons list to evaluate the factors you are considering in making a decision.
- If you decide to work towards your goals or future plans, tell your loved one first.

IN CONCLUSION

Thank you for reading this book and making it to the end! Even if you only selected chapters that seemed more relevant to you, you are demonstrating a desire to help someone you love and they are lucky to have you in their lives. You are not perfect – nobody is – and your responses may not always be perfect. BUT YOU CARE, and that is an amazing starting place. Sometimes, in the midst of a problem, people cannot appreciate the help and support they have. This is not because they don't care or are too selfish; it is because the anxiety problem is pervasive and at times so overwhelming that people can't see beyond the anxiety. It means so much to have someone on your team (even if it is at times conflictual and stressful) when you are suffering from an anxiety or obsessional problem, so on behalf of your loved ones, THANK YOU.

I truly hope that you have found this book helpful and it has given you some ideas of how to approach your current situation and help manage your loved one's anxiety problem. As the family, partners and friends of someone with an anxiety problem, you are integral in their journey to better health. Speaking on behalf of all the mental health professionals, we need you and depend on your input in helping your loved one. You are the cheerleaders, the carers, the financiers, the realists, the supporters, the chauffeurs, the chefs, the babysitters, the co-therapists, and many other important roles in your loved one's life. On top of that, you also have your own life and other family members to look after. Your tireless commitment to your loved one is inspirational and a reminder of the immense value in human relationships.

It is not your fault that your loved one is suffering this way, nor are you responsible for making them better. You can give them all the therapy, medication and opportunity to get better, but they will only make progress if they choose to actively engage in treatments. So, understand what you can do to help them in this process and know it is only your loved one who can take the steps to recovery. If your loved one had a physical health problem – a disease, injury or illness – you would be in a similar position. The problem is that with mental health problems your loved one may look the same and be physically able to do things, but it can be hard to remember that they are indeed suffering from poor health. But just like with medical problems, people can choose to do things to make themselves healthier, to live a different life and make the best of their situations.

Try to remember who your loved one is despite the anxiety problem. The anxiety problem can mask a lot of the qualities, values and personality traits in people. But your loved one is still there, so please find a way to "see" them again and the significance they bring to your life. Human relationships are complex at the best of times, and your loved one's anxiety problem is adding another dimension into your relationship. It might be a real test of your relationship, and if your loved one recovers, you will both find strength in the journey it took to get here.

Many relationship problems are caused by poor communication. Before blaming the anxiety problem for relationship woes, it is worth considering how you and your loved one deal with conflict and talk about difficult issues. Life will always throw up tricky situations and disagreements, so learning to communicate better is essential for a strong and healthy relationship. Whilst not all relationships withstand the pressure that an anxiety or obsessional problem brings, many do and people find that the anxiety problem is just another aspect of a multifaceted relationship. And if your relationship does not continue, the anxiety problem will only be part of the reason the relationship ended.

Remember, always, to prioritise your own wellbeing and that of your family. You can only be the best carer and supporter of your loved one when you have good mental health and wellbeing. You need to spend some time on yourself and give yourself a chance to enjoy life.

When someone you love has a health problem – whether it is mental health or physical health – you naturally change your routines and behaviour to assist them. Unfortunately, in the case of anxiety and obsessional problems, this change usually becomes one of the things that contributes to the problem. Once you have figured out what it is that you are doing that is unhelpful for your loved one – and what has prevented you from working towards your own goals and having good mental and physical health – you will be motivated to change these responses and develop a blueprint for a different future for yourself and your loved one.

There are excellent treatment options available for your loved one and for yourself too if you are suffering from anxiety or depression. There is ongoing research and clinical trials looking at best treatment methods for anxiety and obsessional disorders and we are constantly finding out new information that gives us better understanding of these problems. You can be creative with your loved one in how you access good treatments, and just because one did not work in the past, does not mean another won't, so try again.

And finally, stay hopeful. It is worth remembering that things do not stay the same. As time moves on, so does life. It is impossible for things to stay the same – even if it at times life feels very repetitive. Change will happen in some direction and whether things get worse or they improve, at least it will be different. Change is usually preceded by some disruption – it could be your loved one's mental health deteriorating, the arrival of a new family member, a change in working situations, health problems, or moving to a new place to live. It could be very hard, or it may be an exciting change accompanied with minor distress. Whatever it is, change will happen, and this period of your life is impermanent, as are all moments in life. Things can, and will, be different.

ENDNOTES

i   Bandelow, B., & Michaelis, S. (2015). Epidemiology of Anxiety Disorders in the 21st Century. *Dialogues in Clinical Neuroscience*, 17(3): 327–335;
Ruscio, A. M., Stein, D. J., Chiu, W. T., & Kessler, R. C. (2010). The Epidemiology of Obsessive-Compulsive Disorder in the National Comorbidity Survey Replication. *Molecular Psychiatry*, 15(1): 53–63.

ii   Olatunji, B.O., Cisler, J.M., & Tolin, D.F. (2010). A Meta-analysis of the Influence of Comorbidity on Treatment Outcome in the Anxiety Disorders. *Clinical Psychology Review,* 30(6): 642–54.

iii   Marin, M.F., Lord, C., Andrews, J., Juster, R.P., Sindi, S., Arsenault-Lapierre, G., Fiocco, A.J., & Lupien, S. (2011). Chronic Stress, Cognitive Functioning and Mental Health. *Neurobiology of Learning and Memory*, 96: 583–95.

iv   Baxter, A., Scott, K., Vos, T., & Whiteford, H. (2013). Global Prevalence of Anxiety Disorders: A Systematic Review and Meta-Regression. *Psychological Medicine*, 43(5): 897–910;
Somers, J. M., Goldner, E. M., Waraich, P., & Hsu, L. (2006). Prevalence and Incidence Studies of Anxiety Disorders: A Systematic Review of the Literature. *The Canadian Journal of Psychiatry*, 51(2): 100–113.

v   American Psychiatric Association. (2013). *Diagnostic and Statistical Manual of Mental Disorders* (5th ed.). Arlington, VA: American Psychiatric Publishing.

vi American Psychiatric Association. (2013). *Diagnostic and Statistical Manual of Mental Disorders* (5th ed.). Arlington, VA: American Psychiatric Publishing.

vii Kessler, R.C., Chiu, W.T., Demler, O., Walters, E.E. (2005). Prevalence, Severity, and Comorbidity of 12-Month DSM-IV Disorders in the National Comorbidity Survey Replication. *Archives of General Psychiatry,* 62(6): 617–627.

viii Wittchen, H.U., Gloster, A.T., Beesdo-Baum, K., Fava, G.A., Craske, M.G. (2010). Agoraphobia: A Review of the Diagnostic Classificatory Position and Criteria. *Depression and Anxiety.* 27(2):113–33;
Beesdo-Baum, K., Knappe, S., Pine, D. (2009). Anxiety and Anxiety Disorders in Children and Adolescents: Developmental Issues and Implications for DSM-IV. *Psychiatry Clinics of North America* 32: 483–524.

ix American Psychiatric Association. (2013). *Diagnostic and Statistical Manual of Mental Disorders* (5th ed.). Arlington, VA: American Psychiatric Publishing.

x Salkovskis, P. M. (1985). Obsessional-Compulsive Problems: A Cognitive Behavioural Analysis. *Behaviour Research and Therapy*, 23(5): 571–83.

xi American Psychiatric Association. (2013). *Diagnostic and Statistical Manual of Mental Disorders* (5th ed.). Washington, DC: American Psychiatric Association.

xii American Psychiatric Association. (2013). *Diagnostic and Statistical Manual of Mental Disorders* (5th ed.). Washington, DC: American Psychiatric Association.

xiii Shafran, R., Thordarson, D. S., & Rachman, S. (1996). Thought-Action Fusion in Obsessive Compulsive Disorder. *Journal of Anxiety Disorders*, 10(5): 379–91.

xiv Salkovskis, P. M., Wroe, A. L., Gledhill, A., Morrison, N., Forrester, E., Richards, C. & Thorpe, S. (2000). Responsibility Attitudes and Interpretations are Characteristic of Obsessive Compulsive Disorder. *Behaviour Research and Therapy*, 38(4): 347–72.

xv   Kumar, V., Sattar, Y., Bseiso, A., Khan, S., & Rutkofsky, I. H. (2017). The Effectiveness of Internet-Based Cognitive Behavioral Therapy in Treatment of Psychiatric Disorders. *Cureus*, 9(8).

xvi   NICE. (2005). Obsessive-compulsive disorder and body dysmorphic disorder: treatment. Retrieved from www.nice. org.uk/guidance/cg31 [Accessed 03.09.19].

xvii There is emerging research that this new therapy protocol could be as effective as CBT, although studies are limited at this stage. **NICE** (2013). Social anxiety disorder: recognition, assessment and treatment Clinical guideline [CG159] Retrieved from https://www.nice.org.uk/guidance/cg159 [Accessed 04.09.19].

xviii Tyrer, P., & Tyrer, H. (2018). Health Anxiety: Detection and Treatment. *BJPsych Advances*, 24(1): 66–72.

xix   Hedman, E., Andersson, G., & Andersson, E., et al. (2011). Internet-based Cognitive Behavioural Therapy for Severe Health Anxiety: Randomised Controlled Trial. *British Journal of Psychiatry*, 198(3): 230–6;
Hedman, E., Axelsson, E., Görling, A., et al. (2014). Internet-delivered Exposure-based Cognitive Behavioural Therapy and Behavioural stress management for severe health anxiety: randomised controlled trial. *British Journal of Psychiatry*, 205(4): 307–1.

xx   Arkowitz, H., & Westra, H.A. (2004). Integrating Motivational Interviewing and Cognitive Behavioral Therapy in the Treatment of Depression and Anxiety. *Journal of Cognitive Psychotherapy*, 18(4): 337–350;
Westra, H.A., Arkowitz, H., & Dozois., HJ. (2009). Adding a Motivational Interviewing Pretreatment to Cognitive Behavioral Therapy for Generalized Anxiety Disorder: A Preliminary Randomized Controlled Trial. *Journal of Anxiety Disorders*, 23(8): 1106–17.

xxi   *Cambridge Academic Content Dictionary*, 2017. UK: Cambridge
       University Press.
xxii   Veale, D. (2009). Cognitive Behaviour Therapy for a
       Specific Phobia of Vomiting. *The Cognitive Behaviour
       Therapist*, 2(4), 272–288.
xxiii Öst, L.G. (1987). Applied Relaxation: Description
       of a Coping Technique and Review of Controlled
       Studies. *Behaviour Research and Therapy*, 25(5): 397–409.
xxiv   Mosely, M. (2017). *Clever Guts Diet*. UK: Short Books Ltd.
xxv   Ohayon, M. et al. (2017). National Sleep Foundation's
       Sleep Quality Recommendations: First Report. *Sleep Health*,
       3(1): 6.
xxvi   Baumeister, R. F. & Leary, M. R. (1995). The Need
       to Belong: Desire for Interpersonal Attachments as a
       Fundamental Human Motivation. *Psychology Bulletin*, 117(3):
       497–529.
xxvii Verplanken, B., Fisher, N. (2014). Habitual Worrying and
       Benefits of Mindfulness. *Mindfulness*, 5(5): 566–573.
xxviii World Health Organization (2018). Depression.
       Retrieved from www.who.int/news-room/fact-sheets/
       detail/depression. [Accessed 14.08.19].
xxix   American Psychiatric Association. (2013). *Diagnostic and
       Statistical Manual of Mental Disorders* (5th ed.). Arlington, VA:
       American Psychiatric Publishing.
xxx   American Psychiatric Association. (2013). *Diagnostic and
       Statistical Manual of Mental Disorders* (5th ed.). Arlington, VA:
       American Psychiatric Publishing.
xxxi   Dimidjian, S., Hollon, S. D., Dobson, K. S., Schmaling,
       K. B., Kohlenberg, R. J., Addis, M. E., and Atkins, D.
       C. (2006). Randomized Trial of Behavioral Activation,
       Cognitive Therapy, and Antidepressant Medication in the
       Acute Treatment of Adults with Major Depression. *Journal
       of Consulting and Clinical Psychology*, 74(4): 658.

xxxii   Dimidjian, S., Hollon, S. D., Dobson, K. S., Schmaling, K. B., Kohlenberg, R. J., Addis, M. E., and Atkins, D. C. (2006). Randomized trial of Behavioral Activation, Cognitive Therapy, and Antidepressant Medication in the Acute Treatment of Adults with Major Depression. *Journal of Consulting and Clinical Psychology*, 74(4): 658.

ACKNOWLEDGEMENTS

Thank you to my family, my husband and children, for your patience and support whilst I was writing this book.

NOTE/DISCLAIMER

Trigger encourages diversity and different viewpoints, however, all views, thoughts, and opinions expressed in this book are the author's own and are not necessarily representative of Trigger as an organisation.

All material in this book is set out in good faith for general guidance and no liability can be accepted for loss or expense incurred in following the information given. In particular this book is not intended to replace expert medical or psychiatric advice. It is intended for informational purposes only and for your own personal use and guidance. It is not intended to diagnose, treat or act as a substitute for professional medical advice.

ABOUT TRIGGER PUBLISHING

Trigger is a leading independent altruistic global publisher devoted to opening up conversations about mental health and wellbeing. We share uplifting and inspirational mental health stories, publish advice-driven books by highly qualified clinicians for those in recovery and produce wellbeing books that will help you to live your life with greater meaning and clarity.

Founder Adam Shaw, mental health advocate and philanthropist, established the company with leading psychologist Lauren Callaghan, whilst in recovery from serious mental health issues. Their aim was to publish books which provided advice and support to anyone suffering with mental illness by sharing uplifting and inspiring stories from real life survivors, combined with expert advice on practical recovery techniques.

Since then, Trigger has expanded to produce books on a wide range of topics surrounding mental health and wellness, as well as launching *Upside Down*, its children's list, which encourages open conversation around mental health from a young age.

We want to help you to not just survive but thrive – one book at a time.

Find out more about Trigger Publishing by visiting our website:triggerpublishing.com or join us on:

Twitter @TriggerPub

Facebook @TriggerPub

Instagram @TriggerPub

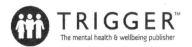

ABOUT SHAW MIND

A proportion of profits from the sale of all Trigger books go to their sister charity, Shaw Mind, also founded by Adam Shaw and Lauren Callaghan. The charity aims to ensure that everyone has access to mental health resources whenever they need them.

You can find out more about the work that Shaw Mind do by visiting their website: shawmindfoundation.org or joining them on
Twitter: @Shaw_Mind
Instagram: @Shaw_Mind
LinkedIn: @shaw-mind
FB: @shawmindUK

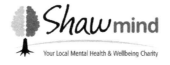

Your Local Mental Health & Wellbeing Charity